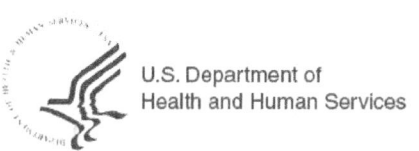

U.S. Department of
Health and Human Services

Physical Activity Guidelines for Americans Midcourse Report

Strategies to Increase Physical Activity Among Youth

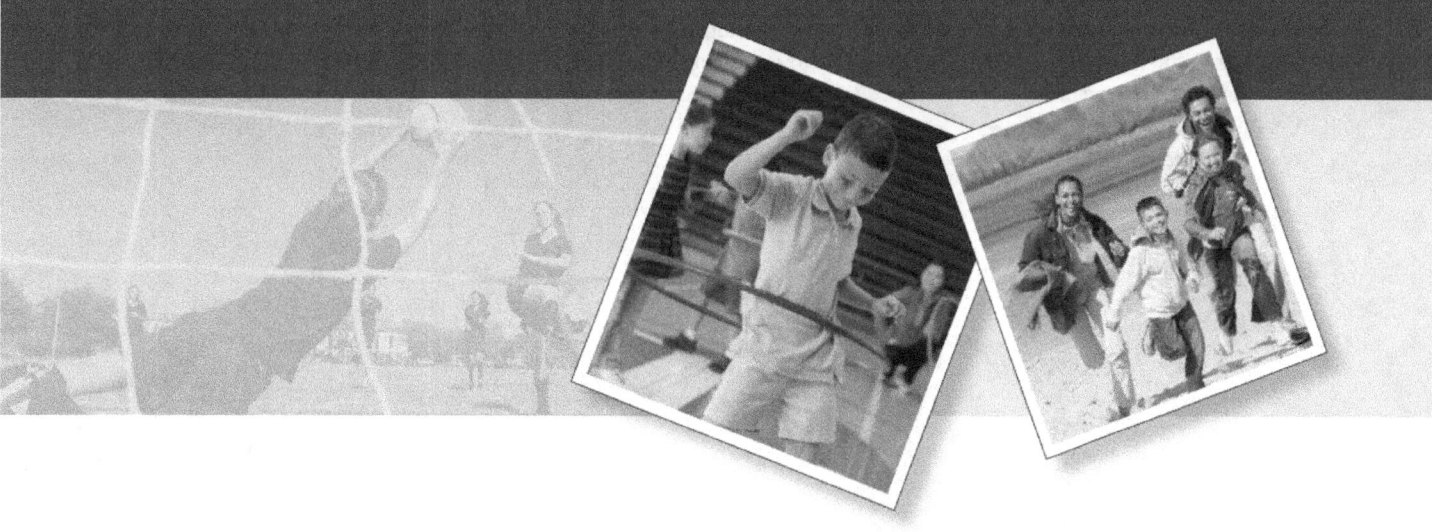

www.health.gov/paguidelines

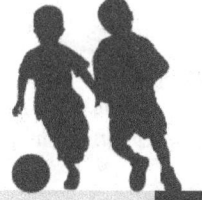

Suggested citation: Physical Activity Guidelines for Americans Midcourse Report Subcommittee of the President's Council on Fitness, Sports & Nutrition. *Physical Activity Guidelines for Americans Midcourse Report: Strategies to Increase Physical Activity Among Youth*. Washington, DC: U.S. Department of Health and Human Services, 2012.

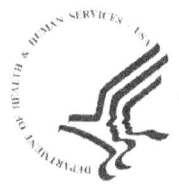

December 31, 2012

The Honorable Kathleen Sebelius
Secretary of Health and Human Services
200 Independence Avenue, S.W.
Washington, D.C. 20201

Dear Secretary Sebelius,

On behalf of the President's Council on Fitness, Sports & Nutrition (PCFSN) and the entire Physical Activity Guidelines Midcourse Report Subcommittee, we are very pleased to submit the *Physical Activity Guidelines for Americans Midcourse Report: Strategies to Increase Physical Activity Among Youth.*

With your approval, a subcommittee of the PCFSN comprised of experts in physical activity was convened to examine the evidence related to strategies to increase physical activity among children and adolescents. The youth population was chosen because this is a time when lifelong physical activity habits can be initiated and fostered. This report documents the findings of this review and presents recommendations on implementation strategies to help young Americans increase physical activity across a variety of settings.

It is not the intent of this report to change recommendations for the type and amount of physical activity for this age group as presented in the *Physical Activity Guidelines for Americans.* Rather, this report highlights physical activity interventions taking place in a variety of settings that were identified through a review-of-reviews. Within the report, evidence-based practices, emerging evidence, and opportunities for additional research are presented.

The Guidelines have been used to inform policies and procedures across the federal government and within communities. For example, Healthy People 2020 contains objectives specific to meeting and achieving the adult and youth Guidelines. The Guidelines for youth provide the foundation on which First Lady Michelle Obama's *Let's Move!* initiative and the White House Childhood Obesity Task Force Report are built. Similarly, the purpose of the National Physical Activity Plan, released in 2009 as a collaboration between federal, state, and private sectors, is to help more Americans achieve the Guidelines. We anticipate this report will add value to existing policies and procedures by providing recommendations for "next steps" to ensure the rapid and effective development of the next generation of intervention strategies to achieve the Guidelines among youth.

It is important to emphasize that this report could not have been completed without the outstanding support of all the U.S. Department of Health and Human Services (HHS) staff who assisted us throughout the entire process. Special recognition goes to Katrina Butner, who served as the Coordinator for this effort, for her tireless dedication to the successful completion of this project. We also appreciate the support of Don Wright, Richard Olson, and Amber Mosher of the Office of Disease Prevention and Health Promotion (ODPHP) and Shellie Pfohl, Megan Nechanicky, and Jane Wargo of the PCFSN. This report greatly benefits from the expert editing provided by Anne Rodgers, who helped us present information that is useful and readable.

Among our most important findings is that school settings provide a realistic and evidence-based prospect for increasing physical activity among youth. This presents a prime opportunity for federal and state leadership to advance the implementation of quality physical activity programs in the school setting. Other settings, particularly preschools and the built environment, also show great promise and warrant continued research emphasis. Multiple stakeholders, including transportation, urban planning, and public safety, as well as health, have an interest in promoting physical activity among youth, and our findings demonstrate that this goal can be met in a variety of ways.

Please do not hesitate to contact me or any of the subcommittee members if we can be of further service.

Sincerely,

Risa Lavizzo-Mourey, MD, MBA
Chair, Physical Activity Guidelines Midcourse Report Subcommittee
Member, President's Council on Fitness, Sports & Nutrition
President and CEO, Robert Wood Johnson Foundation

Contents

▬▬▬ Physical Activity Guidelines for Americans Midcourse Report Membership iv

▬▬▬ Executive Summary and Key Messages..vii

▬▬▬ 1. Introduction 1

    Current Levels of Physical Activity Among Youth...1

    The 2008 Physical Activity Guidelines for Americans..2

    The Midcourse Report: Building on the Physical Activity Guidelines..3

    Organization of the Report 3

▬▬▬ 2. Methods 5

    Conceptual Framework..5

    Literature Review...6

    Report Development and Review...7

▬▬▬ 3. Results by Intervention Setting..9

    School Setting..9

        Multi-component School-based Interventions..9

        Physical Education..10

        Active Transportation to School 11

        Activity Breaks...12

        School Physical Environment 13

        After-school Interventions..13

    Preschool and Childcare Center Setting...15

    Community Setting..16

        Built Environment..16

        Camps and Youth Organizations...17

        Other Community-based Programs 18

    Family and Home Setting 19

    Primary Health Care Setting...20

▬▬▬ 4. Additional Approaches to Consider..23

    Policy..23

    VERB..25

    Technology-based Approaches..25

    Playing Outdoors..26

▬▬▬ References 28

Physical Activity Guidelines for Americans Midcourse Report Membership

President's Council on Fitness, Sports & Nutrition

Co-Chairs

Drew Brees

Dominique Dawes

Members

Dan Barber

Carl Edwards

Allyson Felix

Jayne Greenberg, EdD

Grant Hill

Billie Jean King

Michelle Kwan

Risa Lavizzo-Mourey, MD, MBA

Cornell McClellan

Stephen McDonough, MD

Chris Paul

Curtis Pride

Donna Richardson Joyner

Ian Smith, MD

Physical Activity Guidelines for Americans Midcourse Report Subcommittee

Chair

Risa Lavizzo-Mourey, MD, MBA
Member, President's Council on Fitness, Sports &
Nutrition
President and CEO, Robert Wood Johnson Foundation

Members

Joan M. Dorn, PhD
Chief, Physical Activity and Health Branch
Division of Nutrition, Physical Activity, and Obesity
Centers for Disease Control and Prevention

Janet E. Fulton, PhD
Lead Epidemiologist
Division of Nutrition, Physical Activity, and Obesity
Centers for Disease Control and Prevention

Kathleen F. Janz, EdD
Professor, Department of Health and Human
Physiology
Department of Epidemiology
University of Iowa

Sarah M. Lee, PhD
Lead Health Scientist
Division of Population Health
Centers for Disease Control and Prevention

Robin A. McKinnon, PhD, MPA
Health Policy Specialist
National Cancer Institute
National Institutes of Health

Russell R. Pate, PhD
Professor, Department of Exercise Science
University of South Carolina

Karin Allor Pfeiffer, PhD
Associate Professor, Department of Kinesiology
Michigan State University

Deborah Rohm Young, PhD
Research Scientist, Department of Research and
Evaluation
Kaiser Permanente Southern California

Richard P. Troiano, PhD
Captain, U.S. Public Health Service
National Cancer Institute
National Institutes of Health

U.S. Department of Health and Human Services Federal Steering Committee

Office of Disease Prevention and Health Promotion

Don Wright, MD, MPH
Deputy Assistant Secretary for Health
Director

Katrina L. Butner, PhD, RD, ACSM CES
Coordinator, Physical Activity Guidelines for Americans
Midcourse Report
Physical Activity and Nutrition Advisor

Amber Mosher, MPH, RD
Prevention Science Fellow

Richard D. Olson, MD, MPH
Director, Prevention Science Division

President's Council on Fitness, Sports & Nutrition

Shellie Y. Pfohl, MS
Executive Director

Megan Nechanicky, MS, RD
Oak Ridge Institute for Science and Education Fellow

Jane D. Wargo, MA
Program Analyst

National Institutes of Health

Richard P. Troiano, PhD
Captain, U.S. Public Health Service
National Cancer Institute
National Institutes of Health

Centers for Disease Control and Prevention

Rosemary Bretthauer-Mueller
Lead Health Communication Specialist
Division of Nutrition, Physical Activity, and Obesity

William H. Dietz, MD, PhD
Former Director
Division of Nutrition, Physical Activity, and Obesity

Joan M. Dorn, PhD
Chief, Physical Activity and Health Branch
Division of Nutrition, Physical Activity, and Obesity

Janet E. Fulton, PhD
Lead Epidemiologist
Division of Nutrition, Physical Activity, and Obesity

Office of the Assistant Secretary for Health

Rosie Henson, MSSW, MPH
Senior Advisor

Penelope Slade-Sawyer, PT, MSW
Rear Admiral, U.S. Public Health Service
Senior Advisor

Literature Review Team: Washington University in St. Louis and Universidad de los Andes

Ross Brownson, PhD
Professor and co-director, Prevention Research Center
in St. Louis
Washington University in St. Louis

Amy A. Eyler, PhD
Prevention Research Center in St. Louis
Assistant Professor, Washington University in St. Louis

Rachel Tabak, PhD
Prevention Research Center in St. Louis
Research Assistant Professor, Washington University

Olga L. Sarmiento, MD, MPH, PhD
Associate Professor
Department of Public Health, School of Medicine
Universidad de los Andes
Bogotá, Colombia

Technical Writer and Editor

Anne Brown Rodgers

Reviewers

William H. Dietz, MD, PhD
Former Director
Division of Nutrition, Physical Activity, and Obesity
Centers for Disease Control and Prevention

James F. Sallis, PhD
Distinguished Professor of Family and Preventive Medicine
Chief, Division of Behavioral Medicine
University of California, San Diego

Dianne S. Ward, PhD
Professor
Department of Nutrition
University of North Carolina

Executive Summary and Key Messages

In response to a desire from both federal and non-federal stakeholders for the *2008 Physical Activity Guidelines for Americans* to be updated on a regular basis, the U.S. Department of Health and Human Services (HHS) Office of Disease Prevention and Health Promotion (ODPHP), the President's Council on Fitness, Sports & Nutrition (PCFSN), the Centers for Disease Control and Prevention (CDC), and the National Institutes of Health (NIH) formed a federal steering group to discuss this issue. Although research and new findings in the realm of physical activity continue to emerge, the group believed that the current *Physical Activity Guidelines for Americans* recommendations would change little if they were updated. Therefore, the steering group recommended a Midcourse Report, which would provide an opportunity for experts to review and highlight a specific topic of importance related to the Guidelines and to communicate findings to the public. The steering group identified "strategies to increase physical activity among youth" as a topic area that would help to inform current practice related to the Guidelines.

Physical Activity Guidelines for Americans Midcourse Report: Strategies to Increase Physical Activity Among Youth is intended to identify interventions that can help increase physical activity in youth across a variety of settings. A subcommittee of the PCFSN comprised of experts in physical activity was convened to examine the evidence and deliver their findings in the Midcourse Report. The subcommittee focused on physical activity in general and did not examine specific types of activity, such as muscle- or bone-strengthening physical activities. The subcommittee also did not consider efforts to reduce sedentary time or screen time. The primary audiences for the report are policymakers, health care and public health professionals, and leaders in the settings covered in the report.

Recognizing that many settings have the potential to increase physical activity among youth, the subcommittee focused on five settings in which physical activity interventions for youth have been studied and evaluated and for which review articles existed: schools, preschool and childcare centers, community, family and home, and primary care. To assess the literature on these settings, the subcommittee and a literature review team from Washington University in St. Louis analyzed findings from review articles using a review-of-reviews approach.

This report discusses the importance of each of the five settings and its relation to youth physical activity, presents a review of and conclusions about the strength of evidence supporting interventions to increase physical activity, and describes research needs. The report also discusses several notable precedents for policy involvement in youth physical activity, describes the potential for policy and programs to further encourage increased physical activity among youth, and discusses other approaches to consider in developing strategies to increase physical activity among youth.

The remainder of this Executive Summary highlights key findings and recommendations from the *Midcourse Report* and discusses overarching needs for future research. Table 1 provides a summary of these findings and research needs.

Key Findings and Recommendations

School Settings Hold a Realistic and Evidence-based Opportunity to Increase Physical Activity Among Youth and Should be a Key Part of a National Strategy to Increase Physical Activity

More than 95 percent of youth are enrolled in schools, and a typical school day lasts approximately 6 to 7 hours, making schools an ideal setting to provide physical activity to students.[1] Sufficient evidence is available to recommend wide implementation of multi-component school-based programs. These types of programs provide enhanced physical education (PE) (e.g., increased lesson time, delivery by well-trained specialists, and instructional practices that provide substantial moderate-to-vigorous physical activity), as well as classroom activity breaks, activity sessions before and/or after school, and active transportation to school.

Similarly, well-designed enhanced PE in and of itself increases physical activity among youth and should be widely implemented in schools. Two additional approaches—activity breaks and commuting to and from school using active transport—show promise and are attractive because they can be implemented in situations where a full multi-component program or enhanced PE may be out of reach. Because the scientific knowledge of what works is still evolving, it is critical that, as a nation, we continue to evaluate the impact of physical activity programs in schools and ensure that effective programs are translated for a variety of audiences and widely disseminated.

Preschool and Childcare Centers That Serve Young Children Are an Important Setting in Which to Enhance Physical Activity

Millions of American children spend much of their day in structured childcare centers. More than 4.2 million young children (about 60% of children ages 3 to 5 who are not attending kindergarten) are enrolled in center-based preschools in the United States,[2] and the evidence suggests that well-designed interventions can increase physical activity among these children. Promising interventions include those that increase time children spend outside, provide portable play equipment (e.g., balls and tricycles) on playgrounds and other play spaces, provide staff with training in the delivery of structured physical activity sessions for children and increase the time allocated for such sessions, and integrate physically active teaching and learning activities.

Changes Involving the Built Environment and Multiple Sectors Are Promising

The built environment includes the physical form of communities including urban design (how a city is designed; its physical appearance and arrangement), land use patterns (how land is used for commercial, residential and other activities), and the transportation system (the facilities and services that link one location to another).[3] Changes to this setting are important

because they offer the potential to increase activity for *all* youth, not only those who elect to participate in specific programs or activities, which may be affected by socioeconomic factors.

Multiple national, state, and local stakeholders play an important role in promoting physical activity in this setting, including those in transportation, urban planning, and public safety, whose primary mission is not physical activity promotion. What has yet to be tested is the added value of including these sectors in comprehensive community interventions for youth physical activity.

To Advance Efforts to Increase Physical Activity Among Youth, Key Research Gaps Should Be Addressed

During the development of this report, several research needs emerged that could be applied to all of the five settings addressed. Currently, reviews of physical activity in youth have limited long-term or longitudinal follow up. Extending research beyond short-term interventions can help determine the sustainability and long-term benefits of increasing physical activity among youth. Additionally, research including a variety of demographic, geographic, health status, racial and ethnic, and socioeconomic status groups would be beneficial in determining how interventions can best be applied to specific populations. Behavioral theories underlying the interventions that yield the strongest effects in youth need further examination.

Several settings reviewed by the subcommittee, including Community, Family and Home, and Primary Care, had limited evidence about specific interventions strategies, but showed promise as an opportunity to engage youth. These settings should be highlighted as priority areas for research to better understand how interventions can be applied in both specific areas and across multiple settings to increase opportunities for physical activity.

Finally, most policy-relevant research related to youth physical activity is cross-sectional, showing associations but not permitting causal connections between the policies and programs to be drawn. In the future, longitudinal assessments and rigorous evaluation of policies and programs related to youth physical activity are particularly high priorities.

Table 1. Summary of Findings and Next Steps for Research

Setting and Strength of Evidence*	Strategies to Increase Physical Activity Among Youth	Next Steps for Research
School Setting		
Multi-component *Sufficient*	• Provide enhanced physical education (PE) that increases lesson time, is delivered by well-trained specialists, and emphasizes instructional practices that provide substantial moderate-to-vigorous physical activity. • Provide classroom activity breaks. • Develop activity sessions before and/or after school, including active transportation. • Build behavioral skills. • Provide after-school activity space and equipment.	• Evaluate the translation and dissemination of effective interventions, particularly in the multi-component and PE areas, where sufficient evidence indicates that school programs increase physical activity among youth. • Determine the specific strategies that contribute importantly to the success of multi-component interventions. • Determine specific approaches with the greatest effectiveness for increasing activity transportation to school (e.g., walking school bus). • Examine the effectiveness of approaches to increase physical activity during break times already structured into the school day (e.g., recess) versus other planned times, or the optimal combination of both. • Examine intervention effects on overall daily and weekly physical activity levels. • Conduct intervention studies with long-term follow-up measures. • Conduct intervention studies with robust process evaluation protocols, in addition to examining implementation and sustainability. • Compare intervention effects across race, ethnicity, and socioeconomic groups.
Physical Education *Sufficient*	• Develop and implement a well-designed PE curriculum. • Enhance instructional practices to provide substantial moderate-to-vigorous physical activity. • Provide teachers with appropriate training.	
Active Transportation *Suggestive*	• Involve school personnel in intervention efforts. • Educate and encourage parents to participate with their children in active transportation to school.	
Activity Breaks *Emerging*	• Add short bouts of physical activity to existing classroom activities. • Encourage activity during recess, lunch, and other break periods. • Promote environmental or systems change approaches, such as providing physical activity and game equipment, teacher training, and organized physical activity during breaks before and after school.	
School Physical Environment *Insufficient*	Not applicable	
After School *Insufficient*	Not applicable	

*Table 2, p. 8, provides details on the criteria used to determine the strength of evidence.

Table 1. Summary of Findings and Next Steps for Research (continued)

Setting and Strength of Evidence*	Strategies to Increase Physical Activity Among Youth	Next Steps for Research
Preschool and Childcare Center Setting		
Suggestive	• Provide portable play equipment on playgrounds and other play spaces. • Provide staff with training in the delivery of structured physical activity sessions for children and increase the time allocated for such sessions. • Integrate physically active teaching and learning activities into pre-academic instructional routines. • Increase time that children spend outside.	• Conduct longitudinal, observational studies with rigorous measures. • Examine specific strategies to promote physical activity in the childcare setting. • Conduct policy research to examine the effects of state and institutional policy innovations. • Examine the effect of the center physical environment on child physical activity. • Investigate center-based interventions that involve parents and activities at home. • Compare intervention effects across race, ethnicity, and socioeconomic groups.
Community Setting		
Built Environment *Suggestive*	• Improve the land-use mix to increase the number of walkable and bikeable destinations in neighborhoods. • Increase residential density so that people can use methods other than driving to reach the places they need or want to visit. • Implement traffic-calming measures, such as traffic circles and speedbumps. • Increase access to, density of, and proximity to parks and recreation facilities. • Improve walking and biking infrastructure, such as sidewalks, multi-use trails, and bike lanes. • Increase walkability of communities. • Improve pedestrian safety structures, such as traffic lights. • Increase vegetation, such as trees along streets. • Decrease traffic speed and volume to encourage walking and biking for transportation. • Reduce incivilities and disorders, such as litter and vacant or poorly-maintained lots.	• Conduct studies with longer intervention periods and long-term follow up. • Conduct quasi-experimental evaluation research on the built environment and youth physical activity, taking advantage of "natural experiments" (i.e., environmental changes implemented by policymakers and/or others). • Evaluate the effects of built environment changes on adolescent physical activity. • Assess the effect of neighborhood crime-related safety on youth physical activity. • Develop methods to improve attendance in the programs and interventions under study. • Examine ways to convert summer camp activity into habitual activity. • Examine the role of "location in the community," particularly distance from school or home, on participation and adherence. • Compare intervention effects across race, ethnicity, and socioeconomic groups.
Camps and Youth Organizations *Insufficient*	Not applicable	

*Table 2, p. 8, provides details on the criteria used to determine the strength of evidence.

Table 1. Summary of Findings and Next Steps for Research (continued)

Setting and Strength of Evidence*	Strategies to Increase Physical Activity Among Youth	Next Steps for Research
Community Setting (continued)		
Other Community Programs *Insufficient*	Not applicable	
Family and Home Setting		
Insufficient	Not applicable	• Conduct observational studies to examine the relevance of family and home-based strategies throughout childhood and adolescence. • Conduct longitudinal, observational studies to delineate which components of family life influence children's physical activity behavior. • Test specific strategies that engage parents and other family members in promoting physical activity in the home setting. • Test specific strategies that enrich the home environment to favor activity over sedentary pursuits. • Compare intervention effects across race, ethnicity, and socioeconomic groups.
Primary Care Setting		
Insufficient	Not applicable	• Conduct randomized, controlled studies of the effectiveness of primary care counseling on physical activity behavior. • Identify the optimal intensity and delivery mode of primary care physical activity interventions. • Consider the utility of interventions that combine primary care counseling with referral and integration into community youth-focused programs. • Identify the optimal age range for effective interventions in primary care settings, as well as intervention effects in normal weight as well as overweight or obese youth. • Examine strategies to promote physical activity in different primary care settings, including integrated health care, fee-for-service, and community clinics. • Conduct cost-effectiveness research after effective interventions have been identified. • Compare intervention effects across race, ethnicity, and socioeconomic groups.

*Table 2, p. 8, provides details on the criteria used to determine the strength of evidence.

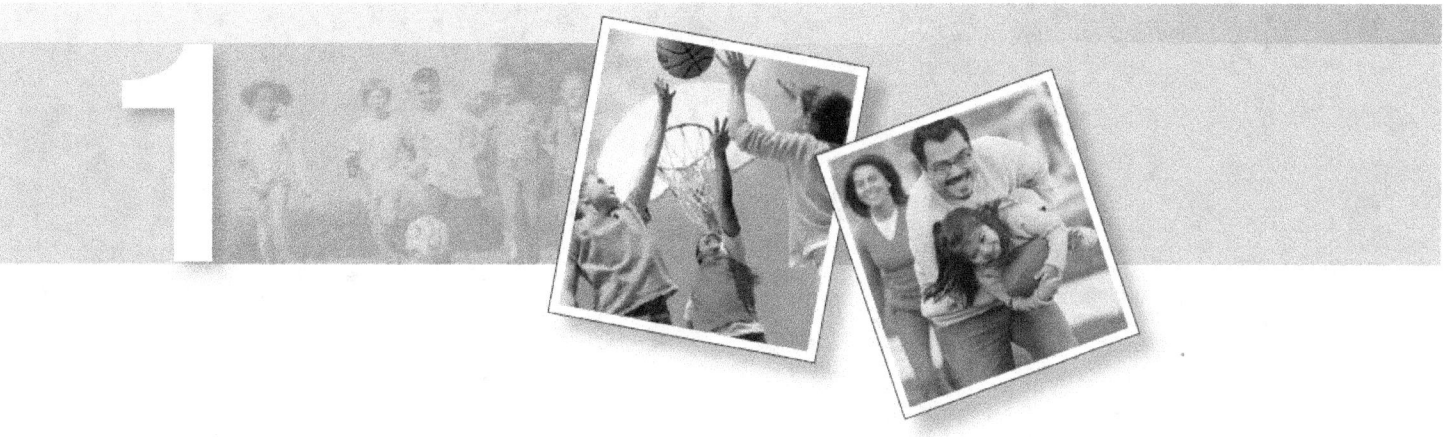

Introduction

Regular physical activity in children and adolescents promotes health and fitness.[4] Compared to those who are inactive, physically active youth have higher levels of cardiorespiratory fitness and stronger muscles. They also typically have lower body fatness. Their bones are stronger and they may have reduced symptoms of anxiety and depression.

Key Terms

In this report, we use the terms:

- youth to include children ages 3 to 11 and adolescents ages 12 to 17, and

- physical activity to refer to bodily movement that enhances health. It includes moderate-intensity activities, such as skateboarding or softball, and vigorous-intensity activities, such as jumping rope or running.

Youth who are regularly active also have a better chance of a healthy adulthood. In the past, chronic diseases, such as heart disease, hypertension, or type 2 diabetes were rare in youth. However, a growing literature is showing that the incidence of these chronic diseases and their risk factors are now increasing among children and adolescents.[5] Regular physical activity makes it less likely that these risk factors and resulting chronic diseases will develop and more likely that youth will remain healthy as adults.

Current Levels of Physical Activity Among Youth

Despite the importance of regular physical activity in promoting lifelong health and well-being, current evidence shows that levels of physical activity among youth remain low, and that levels of physical activity decline dramatically during adolescence. Opportunities for regular physical activity are limited in many schools; daily PE is provided in only 4 percent of elementary schools, 8 percent of middle schools, and 2 percent of high schools.[6] The 2011 National Youth Risk Behavior Survey (YRBS), which collects self-reported physical activity data from high school students across the United States, found that many youth are not meeting the Guidelines recommendation of 60 minutes of physical activity each day:[7]

- 29 percent of high school students participated in at least 60 minutes per day of physical activity on each of the 7 days before the survey. Boys were more than twice as likely as girls to meet the Guidelines (38% vs. 19%).

- 14 percent of high school students did not participate in 60 or more minutes of any kind of physical activity on any day during the 7 days before the survey.

A separate study of U.S. youth used accelerometers to objectively measure physical activity. This study found that 42 percent of children and only 8 percent of adolescents engaged in moderate- to vigorous-intensity activity on 5 of the past 7 days for at least 60 minutes each day.[8]

- Improves cardiorespiratory fitness.

- Strengthens muscles and bones.

- Helps attain/maintain healthy weight.

- Reduces likelihood of developing risk factors for later diseases, such as high blood cholesterol, high blood pressure, and type 2 diabetes, thus increasing the chances that youth will remain healthy as adults.

- May reduce symptoms of anxiety and depression.

The 2008 Physical Activity Guidelines for Americans

In 2008, the U.S. Department of Health and Human Services (HHS) issued the first comprehensive guidelines on physical activity for individuals ages 6 and older. The *2008 Physical Activity Guidelines for Americans* provide information on the amount, types, and intensity of physical activity needed to achieve health benefits across the lifespan.[9]

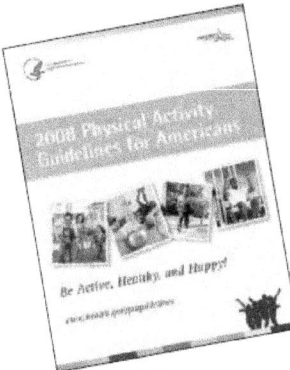

The Guidelines provide physical activity guidance for youth ages 6 to 17 and focus on physical activity beyond the light-intensity activities of daily life, such as walking slowly or lifting light objects. As described in the Guidelines, youth can achieve substantial health benefits by doing moderate- and vigorous-intensity physical activity for periods of time that add up to 60 minutes or more each day. This activity should include aerobic activity as well as age-appropriate muscle- and bone-strengthening activities (see Key Guidelines box, below).

Current science suggests that as with adults, the total amount of physical activity is more important in helping youth achieve health benefits than is any one component (frequency, intensity, or duration) or specific mix of activities (aerobic [e.g., tag, bike riding], muscle-strengthening [e.g., push-ups, climbing trees], or bone strengthening [e.g., hopscotch, tennis]).

Parents and other adults who work with or care for youth should be familiar with the Guidelines, as adults play an important role in providing age-appropriate opportunities for physical activity. They need to foster active play in children and encourage sustained and structured activity in adolescents. In doing so, adults help lay an important foundation for lifelong health, for youth who grow up being physically active are more likely to be active adults.[9]

The Midcourse Report: Building on the Physical Activity Guidelines

In response to a desire from both federal and non-federal stakeholders for the *Physical Activity Guidelines for Americans* to be updated on a regular basis, a federal steering group including representatives from the HHS Office of Disease Prevention and Health Promotion (ODPHP), the President's Council on Fitness, Sports & Nutrition (PCFSN), the Centers for Disease Control and Prevention (CDC), and the National Institutes of Health (NIH) was formed to discuss this issue. Although research and new findings in the realm of physical activity continue to emerge, the group believed that the current Guidelines recommendations would change little if they were updated. Therefore, the steering group recommended a Midcourse Report, which would provide an opportunity for experts to review and highlight a specific topic of importance related to the Guidelines and to communicate findings to the public. With expertise from the PCFSN Science Board and coordination by the ODPHP and PCFSN staff, the steering group identified "strategies to increase physical activity among youth" as a topic area that would help to inform current practice related to the Guidelines.

A subcommittee of the PCFSN was convened in spring 2012 with the approval of HHS Secretary Kathleen Sebelius and Assistant Secretary for Health, Dr. Howard Koh. The subcommittee was comprised of experts in school- and community-based interventions, policy, exercise physiology, epidemiology, measurement/quantification and assessment of physical activity, childhood obesity, public health, and environmental influences on physical activity and was chaired by President's Council Member, Dr. Risa Lavizzo-Mourey. The ODPHP was responsible for coordinating the subcommittee's work.

The subcommittee was asked to review the evidence on strategies to increase youth physical activity and make recommendations. It conducted its work through biweekly conference calls and three in-person meetings held in May, August, and October, 2012. The subcommittee's findings and recommendations are summarized here in the *Physical Activity Guidelines for Americans Midcourse Report: Strategies to Increase Physical Activity Among Youth.*

The *Midcourse Report* is intended to identify interventions that can help increase physical activity in youth across a variety of settings. The subcommittee focused on physical activity in general and did not examine specific types of activity, such as muscle- or bone-strengthening physical activities. The subcommittee also did not consider efforts to reduce sedentary time or screen time. The primary audiences for the report are policymakers, health care and public health professionals, and leaders in the settings covered in the report.

Even though the *2008 Physical Activity Guidelines for Americans* does not include specific recommendations for children younger than age 6, the subcommittee expanded its review to include children ages 3 to 5. This decision was made in light of the fact that physical activity for young children is necessary for healthy growth and development.[9] The environments in which young children spend their days are often less structured than the formal school environments of later childhood and adolescence, thus providing opportunities for the free play and unstructured physical activity that are important for this age group. The subcommittee's consideration of this young age group also is consistent with the recommendations of the Institute of Medicine's 2011 report *Early Childhood Obesity Prevention Policies*[10] and the recommendations of several countries, including Australia and the United Kingdom, that have developed physical activity guidelines for infants and young children.[11-13]

Organization of the Report

The *Midcourse Report* consists of three major components. The first component, which includes the Introduction and Methods sections, describes the background and context for the *Report* and the process by which the subcommittee reviewed the evidence and developed its recommendations.

The second component, Results by Intervention Setting, focuses on five settings that are central to the lives of youth. Each section within this component discusses the importance of the setting and its relationship to youth physical activity, presents a review of and conclusions about the strength of evidence supporting interventions to increase physical activity, and describes research needs. A third component, Additional Approaches to Consider, discusses several notable precedents for policy involvement in youth physical activity and describes the potential for policy and programs to further encourage increased physical activity among youth.

This component also discusses other approaches to consider in developing strategies to increase physical activity among youth, including building on lessons learned from the VERB™ campaign; incorporating the interests, characteristics, and social media habits of today's youth in future physical activity interventions; and emphasizing tried-and-true methods, such as playing outdoors.

The *Report* contains a number of terms important to physical activity and health. Definitions of these terms can be found in the *2008 Physical Activity Guidelines for Americans* Glossary (http://www.health.gov/paguidelines/guidelines/glossary.aspx).

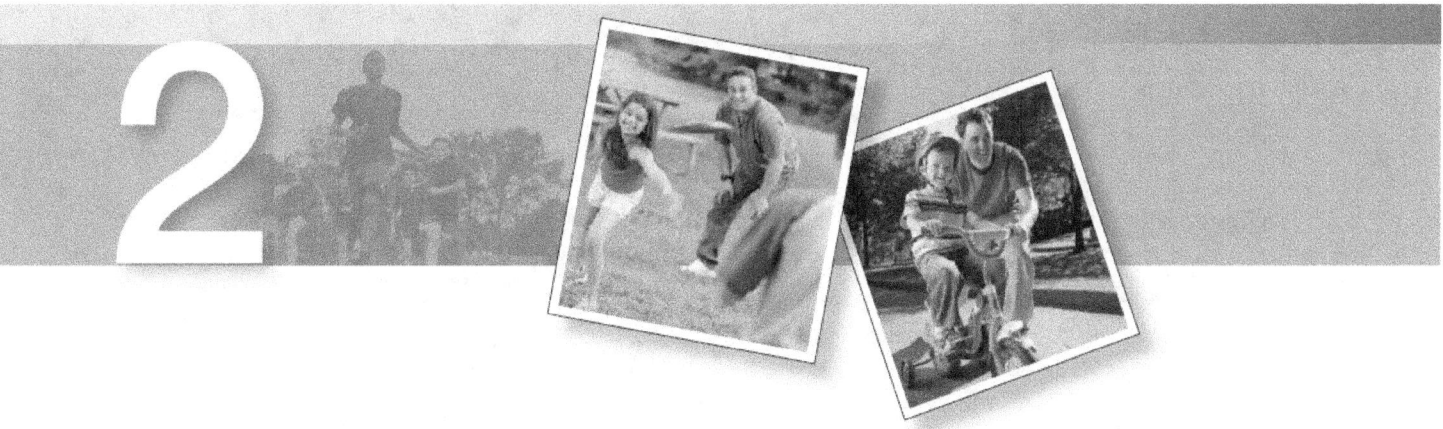

Methods

The CDC contracted with Washington University researchers at the Prevention Research Center (PRC) in St. Louis to conduct the literature review for the *Physical Activity Guidelines for Americans Midcourse Report*. A team from the PRC used Washington University library services to carry out the literature review, which was coordinated by the ODPHP and the CDC Division of Nutrition, Physical Activity, and Obesity, Physical Activity and Health Branch. The subcommittee and the PRC team together determined that the literature review team would use a review-of-reviews approach to assess the current literature on interventions to increase physical activity in youth across the five selected settings. When more than one narrative or systematic review has been published, the use of this methodology facilitates the examination and comparison of intervention strategies and results because it allows for the translation and synthesis of knowledge across multiple reviews that include multiple studies. Because the PRC team had used the review-of-reviews approach previously, they took the lead in determining the operational plan and literature review process, with regular consultation from the subcommittee. A representative from the PRC team participated in the subcommittee's meetings to provide regular updates on the literature review process, and to answer subcommittee questions about findings from the literature.

Several limitations of our review are worth noting. First, by its nature, a review-of-reviews includes only work published in peer-reviewed publications. Consequently, some relevant documents, such as those by the Institute of Medicine (IOM) and National Institute for Health and Clinical Excellence (NICE), and those found in the grey literature, such as policy documents, were not included. Another drawback is that some areas of research were not included, as they are too new to the scientific literature to have been reviewed. The subcommittee did not use the review-of-reviews method for the section on Additional Approaches to Consider because reviews do not yet exist in these areas. Third, a thorough assessment of the quality of the reviews was not included, as would be conducted in a systematic review. The review-of-reviews approach also precluded an assessment of quality at the individual study level (e.g., taking into account study design and study execution), and the subcommittee did not examine individual studies for their contributions to the findings. Finally, the review-of-reviews methodology did not allow the subcommittee to identify specific theories that could be used to structure potentially effective interventions or to critically evaluate external validity.

Conceptual Framework

The subcommittee used an ecological framework to identify settings where youth live, learn, and play. Recognizing that many settings have potential for increasing physical activity among youth but that evidence across the settings varies, the subcommittee focused on five in which physical activity interventions for youth have been studied and evaluated: schools, preschool and childcare centers, community, family and home, and primary care.

Literature Review

The review-of-reviews process to assess the current level of evidence for physical activity interventions in youth began in summer 2012 and continued through early fall 2012. The basis for the current review-of-reviews was formed by two previously published review-of-reviews.[14, 15] Using the seven-step process described below, the PRC team identified review articles published from January 2001 through July 2012, determined which articles should be included based on inclusion and exclusion criteria developed by the subcommittee, and then abstracted and synthesized the data. A total of 31 reviews containing 910 studies (this number includes some studies that were cited in more than one review) ultimately were included.

Inclusion and Exclusion Criteria for the Review-of-Reviews

Inclusion Criteria

- Youth ages 3–17 years
- English language
- Peer-reviewed literature of intervention studies
- Systematic reviews and meta-analyses
- Reviews published January 2001 through July 2012
- Interventions must measure physical activity as an outcome
- Interventions including technology approaches to promote physical activity
- Primarily healthy population
- Results must be available specifically for children or adolescents

Exclusion Criteria

- Interventions focused on limiting screen time
- Interventions focused on decreasing sedentary behavior
- Interventions focused solely on weight loss
- Review containing only cross-sectional data

A key inclusion criterion was the measurement of physical activity as an intervention outcome. Because physical activity measures must be consistent with the intervention targets, physical activity assessment measures included in the reviews covered by this review-of-reviews were device-based measures, self-report, and direct observations. In cases where a particular aspect of physical activity was the intervention target, self-report measures or direct observation that can identify specific behaviors were deemed to be preferable to device-based measures, which cannot identify behaviors or context.

The literature search and synthesis process involved the following steps:

1. **Select Database(s) Most Likely to Yield the Desired Document Types.** The search for reviews of physical activity interventions in any language was conducted using the following databases: Database of Abstracts of Reviews of Effects (DARE), the Cochrane library, Turning Research Into Practice (TRIP), PubMed (Medline), the American Psychological Association, and National Guidelines Clearinghouse.

2. **Determine Search Parameters and Conduct the Search.** The evidence resources reviewed and abstracted were limited to those published between January 2001 through July 2012, plus articles accepted for publication in English-language, peer-reviewed journals. Search terms included: "physical activity," "interventions," "systematic review," "meta analysis," "child," and "adolescent." The Washington University library system was used to conduct the search.

3. **Screen the Titles and Abstracts to Determine Potential Relevance.** The results were automatically filtered through the databases for date (January 2001 through July 2012) and English language. One reviewer then manually filtered the titles and abstracts for age of the populations in the reviews. Two reviewers examined the databases and included all titles and abstracts that met the inclusion criteria, as well as those for which the applicability of the inclusion criteria could not be determined. These same two reviewers then examined the abstracts for further information regarding inclusion.

4. **Obtain Selected Documents.** The literature review team obtained copies of the complete articles selected through the Washington University library system.

5. **Perform an Initial Synthesis to Determine Inclusion.** Relevant review articles were screened to ensure each document met the inclusion criteria.

6. **Abstract Selected Review Articles and Summarize.** All relevant articles that met the inclusion criteria were summarized and information was abstracted to create detailed evidence tables. These tables included the following information:

   - Methodological information: reference, year of publication, objective, type of review (systematic, narrative), type of studies/methods reviewed (e.g., randomized controlled trial, quasi-experimental design), review methods, number of included studies, year of publication, study populations and settings, independent variables, dependent variables.

   - Intervention information: type of intervention, age group, focus on high-risk population, setting, number of studies, number of children, countries/region of studies.

   - Results: main conclusion, race/ethnic groups and low socioeconomic status group estimates. (Note: Effect size estimates and sufficient information for calculating pooled mean effect sizes were collected but the information was not sufficient to make comparisons across population subgroups.)

   - Information to determine level of evidence: determined in part by type of studies/methods reviewed and assessed as a component of "methodological information."

Using the information contained in the evidence tables, the literature review team then collectively and systematically reviewed physical activity intervention strategies to assess their effectiveness. Emerging intervention strategies were assessed, reviewed, and reported when available, but many were so recent that they had not yet been incorporated into systematic evidence reviews and therefore may not have been included in the *Midcourse Report.*

7. **Synthesize Evidence.** The final step was to synthesize the evidence by setting. To determine the quality, strength, and consistency of the available evidence for each of these settings and sub-topics, the subcommittee reviewed the evidence tables and used the most relevant reviews. The most relevant reviews were those dedicated to the setting (if available), those with sections dedicated to the setting (if available), or those with discussion/conclusions dedicated to the setting. The evidence within each of these settings was then classified into one of the following categories (sufficient, suggestive, insufficient [including emerging or no evidence], or evidence of no effect) developed by the subcommittee using the specific criteria contained in Table 2.

Report Development and Review

Once the literature review was completed, subcommittee members drafted individual sections of the report. The sections were reviewed and discussed by all members of the subcommittee and revised multiple times. The completed draft was reviewed by three leading physical activity experts and made available for public comment from November 9 to December 10, 2012. The subcommittee carefully considered all the comments generated from the external review and public comment process and made a number of changes to the report in response. Many of the comments addressed the need for special attention to disparities, underserved populations, and the built environment. While the subcommittee acknowledges the importance of these issues, the ability to generalize recommendations to all populations and settings is limited by the available data. These limitations underscore the urgent need for additional research, and the research recommendations included here are intended to address this need.

Table 2. Assessing the Strength of Evidence of Reviews

Evidence of effectiveness	Adequate evidence	Consistency across reviews	Addresses methodological issues	Specificity of intervention	# subjects/ sites	#/breadth of studies	Representation	Duration of intervention
Sufficient	Likely/high probability	Likely/high probability	Likely/high probability	Yes	Acceptable	Acceptable	Acceptable	Acceptable
Suggestive	Possibly	Possibly	Possibly	Varies	Acceptable	Acceptable	Acceptable	Acceptable
Insufficient • Emerging evidence • No evidence	Varies	Possibly	Possibly	Varies	Limited	Limited	Limited	Limited
Evidence of no effect	Likely/high probability	Likely/high probability	Likely/high probability	Yes	Acceptable	Acceptable	Acceptable	Acceptable

Definitions

Using the review-of-reviews process, the subcommittee established and defined the following categories of evidence. They found no reviews that fit into the final two categories and therefore made no recommendations about implementation or additional research.

Sufficient: Consistent beneficial effects documented across studies and populations. The subcommittee recommended implementation of these approaches.

Suggestive: Reasonably consistent evidence of effect, but cannot make strong definitive conclusions. The subcommittee recommended implementation and continued research on the impact of these approaches. See the research recommendations in each section.

Insufficient: Do not have enough evidence to make a conclusion. The subcommittee did not recommend implementation. Some of these approaches merit additional research, and recommendations are made in each section.

Emerging evidence: New data, currently being studied, but reviews specific to topic do not yet exist. The subcommittee identified those areas where the technologies and evidence are changing rapidly, thus meriting additional research.

No evidence: Evidence within review articles does not exist in this area.

Evidence of no effect: Consistent lack of effect documented across studies and populations.

3

Results by Intervention Setting

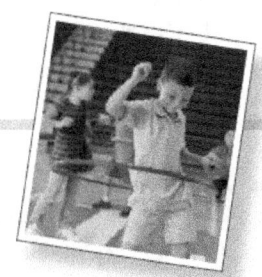

School Setting

More than 55 million children were expected to attend public or private school in the fall of 2012[16] and a typical school day lasts approximately 6 to 7 hours, making schools an ideal setting to provide physical activity to students.[1] School-based physical activity can provide a substantial amount of students' daily physical activity as well as engage them in opportunities to enhance their motor skill development, fitness, and decision making, cooperation, and conflict resolution skills.[17-24] Promoting physical activity in schools has traditionally been a part of the U.S. education system, and schools continue to play a critical role in promoting physical activity. This can occur in a variety of ways, such as through encouraging participation in PE classes, recess and other activity breaks during the school day, active transportation to and from school, sports clubs, intramural and interscholastic programs, and after-school programs.

Schools are a key setting for physical activity interventions also because of a growing body of research focusing on the association between physical activity and academic achievement. These studies indicate that school-based physical activity can improve grades, standardized test scores, cognitive skills, concentration, and attention.[6]

The scientific literature relevant to the schools setting and physical activity in youth describes an array of strategies. For this report, school-related literature is separated into the following areas:

- Multi-component school-based interventions.
- Physical education.
- Active transportation to school.
- Activity breaks.
- School physical environment.
- After-school interventions.

Multi-component School-based Interventions

Multi-component interventions are those in which two or more intervention strategies are concurrently implemented. In the school setting, such interventions have typically been carried out by school staff who interact with interventionists (often university-based). These interventions have usually included a component that aimed to enhance the PE program. Enhancing a PE program is done through increasing physically active time in PE class, adding more PE to the school curriculum, and/or lengthening the PE class time (see the box on Enhanced PE, p. 10). Other strategies include health education, classroom physical activities, enhanced recess, social marketing campaigns, before- and after-school programs, active transportation to school, parent and family involvement, and physical environment enhancements.

Conclusion

Evidence is sufficient that multi-component school-based interventions can increase physical activity during school hours among youth.

Effective strategies include:

- Providing enhanced PE that increases lesson time, is delivered by well-trained specialists, and emphasizes instructional practices that provide substantial moderate-to-vigorous intensity physical activity.

- Providing classroom activity breaks.

- Developing activity sessions before and/or after school, including active transportation.

- Building behavioral skills.

- Providing after-school activity space and equipment.

Supporting Discussion

The majority of the evidence about this setting originates from seven relevant reviews that focused solely on the school setting.[25-31] Findings from these reviews indicate that multi-component interventions with educational, curricular, and environmental components are more effective than are isolated education or curricular components. Successful strategies include intervening over an entire school year, integrating programs into the regular school curriculum, offering enhanced PE as one of the components, providing instruction in the behavioral skills that support adoption and maintenance of physically active lifestyles (e.g., goal setting, building social support), providing educational materials, and involving families. Evidence indicates that offering physical activity breaks and after-school activity space and equipment, as well as increasing time in PE, are effective. The most effective strategies differed by age.[26, 27] For instance, among children, PE combined with activity breaks (e.g., recess, classroom PE breaks) or with family strategies (e.g., engaging parents by sharing written information about physical activity) were most successful.[27] Among adolescents, evidence for including both school and family or community components is strong.[26] Although multi-component school interventions are effective in increasing physical activity during school hours, these interventions are less effective at increasing physical activity outside of school.

Physical Education

PE provides students the opportunity to obtain the knowledge and skills needed to establish and maintain a physically active lifestyle through childhood and adolescence and into adulthood.[32] PE can enhance students' knowledge and skills about why and how they should be physically active,[18, 24] increase participation in physical activity, and increase fitness.[18, 33-38]

Traditionally, PE has been characterized by sports- and performance-based curriculum and instruction. A newer approach—enhanced PE—is characterized by a focus on increasing overall physical activity, particularly moderate-to-vigorous intensity physical activity during PE class.

Enhanced PE

Enhanced PE can increase the amount of time students are active during PE classes as well as increase students' physical fitness levels. Enhanced PE is characterized by the following components:

- Increasing the amount of time students spend in moderate-to-vigorous intensity physical activity during PE lessons.

- Adding more physical education classes to the school curriculum.

- Lengthening the time of existing physical education classes.

- Meeting the physical activity needs of all students, including those with disabilities.

Including activities that are enjoyable for students while emphasizing knowledge and skills that can be used for a lifetime.

Conclusion

Evidence is sufficient that enhanced PE can increase overall physical activity among youth and can increase physical activity time during PE class.

Effective strategies include:

- Developing and implementing a well-designed PE curriculum.

- Enhancing instructional practices to provide substantial moderate-to-vigorous physical activity.

- Providing teachers with appropriate training.

Supporting Discussion

Seven reviews were identified that were either specifically focused on PE or had separate sections about PE.[18, 25, 27, 39-42] Five of the seven reviews did assess the methodological quality of the included studies in the review, while two reviews did not assess methodological quality. Two reviews were broad in scope (i.e., part of a comprehensive school-based intervention review) and included a section on PE.[18, 25] Four reviews evaluated interventions in multiple settings, but had a section on PE.[27, 40-42]

Across the reviews, results indicated that improvements in PE, and therefore in youth physical activity participation, can happen through implementation of strategies either individually or in combination. The overarching PE strategies that were reported to be most effective are changes to the curriculum, selection of lessons to increase physical activity time in PE, and classroom management skills implemented by PE teachers. A well-designed PE curriculum, for example, describes what students should know and be able to do as a result of the PE program, includes lessons that focus on behavior modification and intrinsic motivation, includes lessons focused on keeping students active the majority of class time, and adds fitness and circuit training stations to lesson plans. Enhancing instructional strategies, such as modifying rules of games (e.g., having all students run bases in softball) or substituting less active games with more active ones helps maximize the inclusion of all students in PE. Finally, employing qualified PE teachers

(e.g., certified, licensed, or endorsed to teach PE) and providing teachers with adequate and appropriate training is important to enhancing PE and keeping students in moderate-to-vigorous intensity physical activity for the majority of class time. Training for PE teachers should include strategies for classroom management, how to keep transitions between activities physically active, and how to implement the PE curriculum. The included reviews indicate that these strategies can significantly contribute to a child's overall total moderate-to-vigorous intensity physical activity and increase activity time in PE.

Active Transportation to School

More than 95 percent of youth are enrolled in schools. Thus, addressing active transportation to school has the potential to affect the physical activity of a substantial portion of the youth population. Active transportation to school has been defined as "the use of active means, such as walking and bicycling, to and from school."[43] Active transportation to school has decreased from approximately 41 percent in 1969 to 13 percent in 2001.[44] These falling rates of active transportation to school have prompted policy initiatives, such as Safe Routes to School, and inclusion of active transportation objectives in Healthy People 2020,[45] the 10-year national objectives for improving the health of all Americans. The falling rates also have encouraged researchers to examine and create interventions that address active transportation to school. Active transportation also is influenced by the built environment, which is discussed in more detail in the Community section of this report (see p. 16).

Conclusion

Evidence is suggestive that active transportation to school increases physical activity among youth.

Effective strategies include:

- Involving school personnel in intervention efforts.

- Educating and encouraging parents to participate with their children in active transportation to school.

Supporting Discussion

Three reviews specific to active transportation to school were identified.[43, 46, 47] One included intervention studies,[43] while the others provided cross-sectional evidence. Additionally, four other reviews included active transportation to school as part of their discussion regarding strategies to increase physical activity.[18, 48-50] The existing cross-sectional evidence shows clear associations between active transportation to school and physical activity. On average, the intervention studies show small, but positive, effects.

The one review of interventions included 14 studies specifically focused on active transportation to school.[43] The degree of change in physical activity varied from 3 percent to 64 percent, with nine studies showing trivial or small effect sizes, two showing large effect sizes, and one showing very large effect sizes. Effect size could not be calculated for two studies.

Several different strategies, such as forming walking school buses, providing curricula and resources, and improving safety of school routes by identifying the safest routes, were included across the interventions. Some study designs were weak, so it is difficult to recommend a particular mode or type of programming that works best. However, studies with the greatest effect size indicated that involving school personnel and educating and encouraging parents were important intervention components.[43] Additionally, the walking school bus was implemented in approximately half of the studies showing moderate-to-very large effect size.[43]

Activity Breaks

The school setting can offer opportunities for students to participate in and enjoy physical activity outside of PE class, including recess and physical activity within the classroom. Such opportunities are referred to as activity breaks. Most often, the overarching strategy behind activity breaks has been to establish an environment that promotes regular physical activity throughout the school day. This can occur through regularly scheduled recess and lunch time physical activity or by implementing 5- to 10-minute breaks during classroom time that may or may not include subject matter curriculum.

Conclusion

Evidence is emerging that school-based physical activity breaks can increase physical activity among youth.

Effective strategies include:

- Adding short bouts of physical activity to existing classroom activities.

- Encouraging activity during recess, lunch, and other break periods.

- Promoting environmental or systems change approaches, such as providing physical activity and game equipment, teacher training, and organized physical activity during breaks and before and after school.

Supporting Discussion

Seven relevant reviews were identified.[18, 25, 27, 39-42] Two of the reviews evaluated interventions from many settings and had a section dedicated to activity breaks.[27, 50] Four of the reviews evaluated interventions in multiple settings, but did not have a section dedicated to a review of studies that focused on activity breaks.[30, 31, 39, 51] However, they did include at least one intervention that used activity breaks and they provided some conclusion or discussion about the topic.

Of the two reviews that had a section on activity breaks, interventions incorporated structured physical activity sessions into the school day, added physical activity into usual classroom activities, and used adults to encourage activity during classroom breaks, such as recess or lunch. The four reviews that evaluated interventions in multiple studies did identify that strategies, such as providing game equipment during recess and lunch breaks; organizing physical activities during, before, and after school times; and increasing the availability of physical activity opportunities, combined with other environmental strategies, can increase students' physical activity. However, it is difficult to make conclusions about the isolated impact of physical activity breaks on youth physical activity, given that the reviews included studies of multi-component programs, and activity breaks were only one of many intervention strategies.

School Physical Environment

In recent years, researchers have begun to focus on an ecological perspective that considers environmental factors when examining and designing programs to increase youth physical activity.[52] School physical environment is defined as the physical surroundings affiliated with any given school, including the school's neighborhood and grounds, building design, facilities, and equipment.[53] Although some aspects of school physical environment may be related to the built environment (see p. 16 for more details on physical activity and the built environment), studies of school physical environment often consider other aspects, such as portable equipment and availability of resources. Researchers also often address other aspects of school environment, such as social environment, in their physical activity interventions. The social aspects of the school environment may be important intervention targets, but are not addressed here.

Conclusion

Evidence is insufficient that interventions to modify the school physical environment alone increase physical activity in youth.

Supporting Discussion

A total of 14 reviews were identified. None specifically focused on the school physical environment setting. One review that focused on multiple settings addressed school physical environment separately.[25] Ten reviews included school environment as a single component of multi-component approaches.[17, 27, 30, 40, 52-57] Three other reviews,[24, 26, 49] which focused on multi-component interventions, included school physical environment in their discussions but noted that evidence about this topic is insufficient to draw conclusions.

Intervening on the school environment alone is not typical, in part because of the feasibility and/or cost limitations of changing aspects of the school physical environment, such as building design. In the one review that focused on multiple settings, four studies addressed children, and one addressed adolescents.[25] Three of these five studies were considered relatively

low-quality randomized clinical trials and had limited evidence (children) or inconclusive evidence (adolescents) of school physical environment affecting physical activity. In the 10 reviews that included school physical environment as one component of a multi-component approach, the lack of information made it difficult to separate the effects of the physical environment itself from other components of the intervention.

After-school Interventions

After-school interventions aim to increase physical activity outside of the regular school day. (These types of intervention also are referred to as "out-of-school time" interventions because they can include activities that occur before school.) After-school interventions may be carried out within the school setting or in the community, such as at community centers or YMCAs. Schools and community organizations often collaborate to provide after-school physical activity interventions, such as youth sports.

After-school interventions can be developed and delivered by school staff, teachers, community volunteers, and leaders of community-based after-school programs. They can either be stand-alone programs that solely focus on physical activity or they can be a component of a larger extracurricular or enrichment program.

Conclusion

Evidence is insufficient that promoting physical activity in an after-school setting increases physical activity among youth.

Supporting Discussion

Two narrative reviews[54, 55] and one meta-analysis[56] examined intervention studies that sought to increase youth physical activity in the after-school setting. Three narrative reviews[27, 50, 57] were broader in scope and included the after-school setting as part of an overarching review of interventions to increase youth physical activity. Taken together, the reviews suggest interventions to increase physical activity in the after-school setting may be a promising strategy, although their effectiveness to date has not been shown.[56]

After-school activity intervention programs are generally well-received and enjoyed by youth and parents.[55] The reviews suggest that investigators consider several key implementation strategies in future studies, such as targeting physical activity alone, rather than targeting multiple outcomes, and locating after-school interventions in schools to remove transportation as a barrier.[54]

Next Steps for Research in the School Setting

- Evaluate the translation and dissemination of effective interventions, particularly in the multi-component and PE areas, where sufficient evidence indicates that school programs increase physical activity among youth.

- Determine the specific strategies that contribute importantly to the success of multi-component interventions.

- Determine specific approaches with the greatest effectiveness for increasing active transportation to school (e.g., walking school bus).

- Examine the effectiveness of approaches to increase physical activity during break times already structured into the school day (e.g., recess) versus other planned times, or the optimal combination of both.

- Examine intervention effects on overall daily and weekly physical activity levels.

- Conduct intervention studies with long-term follow-up measures.

- Conduct intervention studies with robust process evaluation protocols, in addition to examining implementation and sustainability.

- Compare intervention effects across race, ethnicity, and socioeconomic groups.

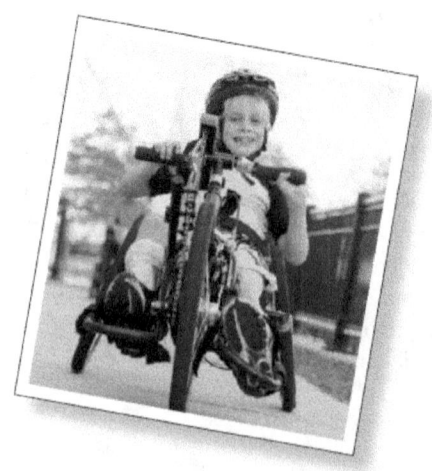

Preschool and Childcare Center Setting

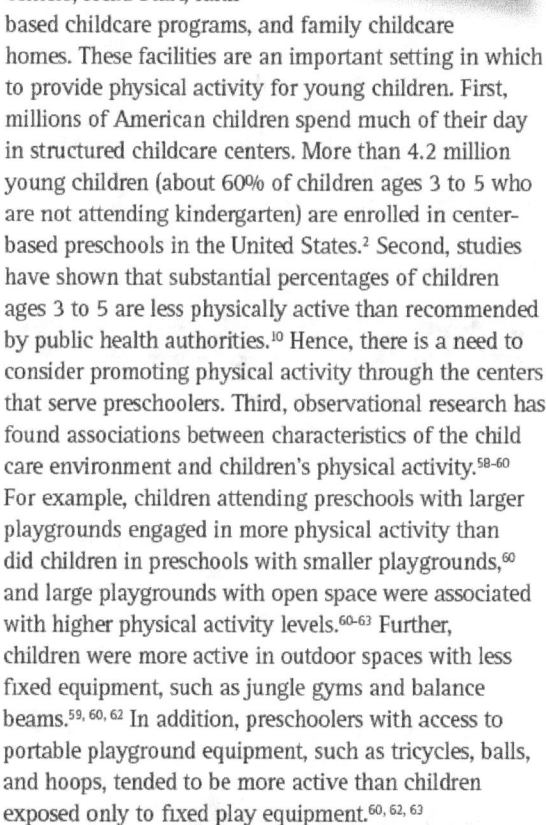

Early care and education centers that serve preschool-aged children include a variety of programs and facilities, such as structured out-of-home preschools and childcare centers, Head Start, faith-based childcare programs, and family childcare homes. These facilities are an important setting in which to provide physical activity for young children. First, millions of American children spend much of their day in structured childcare centers. More than 4.2 million young children (about 60% of children ages 3 to 5 who are not attending kindergarten) are enrolled in center-based preschools in the United States.[2] Second, studies have shown that substantial percentages of children ages 3 to 5 are less physically active than recommended by public health authorities.[10] Hence, there is a need to consider promoting physical activity through the centers that serve preschoolers. Third, observational research has found associations between characteristics of the child care environment and children's physical activity.[58-60] For example, children attending preschools with larger playgrounds engaged in more physical activity than did children in preschools with smaller playgrounds,[60] and large playgrounds with open space were associated with higher physical activity levels.[60-63] Further, children were more active in outdoor spaces with less fixed equipment, such as jungle gyms and balance beams.[59, 60, 62] In addition, preschoolers with access to portable playground equipment, such as tricycles, balls, and hoops, tended to be more active than children exposed only to fixed play equipment.[60, 62, 63]

Conclusion

Evidence is suggestive that interventions to modify the social and/or physical environment in early care and education centers can increase physical activity among young children during the school day.

Strategies, applied independently or collectively, that may increase physical activity include:

- Providing portable play equipment on playgrounds and other play spaces.

Conclusion (continued)

- Providing staff with training in the delivery of structured physical activity sessions for children and increasing the time allocated for such sessions.
- Integrating physically active teaching and learning activities into pre-academic instructional routines.
- Increasing time that children spend outside.

Supporting Discussion

Although eight reviews were identified, the majority of the evidence originates from three reviews that focused solely on the childcare setting.[64-66] Portable play equipment, but not fixed equipment or playground markings, appear more likely to stimulate more physical activity. Teachers' knowledge about physical activity and motor development and their ability to support children's learning and development is important. Therefore, policies promoting structured physical activity also should consider the need for teacher training. Physical activity can and should be integrated into the daily routines and existing curricula of preschools and must not be seen as something that competes with other educational goals. Research also suggests that regularly provided, structured physical activity programs can increase the amount and intensity of physical activity and improve motor skills. However, programs to increase structured physical activity should not be carried out at the expense of children's free play.

Next Steps for Research in the Preschool and Childcare Center Setting

- Conduct longitudinal, observational studies with rigorous measures.
- Examine specific strategies to promote physical activity in the childcare setting.
- Conduct policy research to examine the effects of state and institutional policy innovations.
- Examine the effect of the center physical environment on child physical activity.
- Investigate center-based interventions that involve parents and activities at home.
- Compare intervention effects across race, ethnicity, and socioeconomic groups.

Community Setting

The community setting has enormous potential to increase physical activity in youth by shaping the sociocultural and physical environments where they live, learn, and play. Intervening in community settings can affect activity at the population level, thus potentially providing opportunities and encouragement for *all* youth to be more active.

The Guide to Community Preventive Services[67] defines community as "a group of individuals sharing one or more characteristics such as geographic location (e.g., a neighborhood), culture, age, or a particular risk factor." Consistent with the Community Guide, the broadest possible use of the term "community" was applied while reviewing and summarizing the relevant literature in this area.

The scientific literature relevant to the community setting and physical activity in youth describes an array of strategies, including structural changes to the built environment as well as informational and programmatic interventions conducted in various community locations. For this report, the community-related literature is separated into the following general areas:

- The built environment.

- Programmatic interventions offered in camps and youth organizations.

- Other community-based programs.

After-school programs, often led by community groups, have been described previously in the School setting section of this report (p. 13).

Built Environment

The built environment includes the physical form of communities including urban design (how a city is designed; its physical appearance and arrangement), land use patterns (how land is used for commercial, residential and other activities), and the transportation system (the facilities and services that link one location to another).[3] Changes in this setting are important because they offer the potential to increase activity for all youth, not only those who participate in specific programs or activities, which may be affected by socioeconomic factors. The features of the built environment most relevant to physical activity in youth include parks and recreation facilities, transportation systems, and urban planning aspects, such as sidewalks and local zoning decisions. Research suggests that youth active transportation (i.e., walking or biking to school or other destinations) is influenced by aspects of the built environment, including neighborhood walkability, provision of sidewalks, and reasonable distances for youth to walk or bike to school.[68] (Active transportation to school is addressed in more detail in the School section of this report, see p. 11).

Modifications to the built environment have previously been recommended as a way to increase activity levels in the general population.[40, 67, 69-72] However, few studies have focused on the built environment and its influence on youth activity.[73, 74]

Conclusion

Evidence is suggestive that modifying aspects of the built environment can increase physical activity among youth, particularly:

- Improving the land-use mix to increase the number of walkable and bikeable destinations in neighborhoods.

- Increase residential density so that people can use methods other than driving to reach the places they need or want to visit.

- Implementing traffic-calming measures, such as traffic circles and speed bumps.

Evidence also suggests that changes in the following may increase activity in children:

- Increasing access to, density of, and proximity to parks and recreation facilities.

- Improving walking and biking infrastructure, such as sidewalks, multi-use trails, and bike lanes.

- Increasing walkability (a pattern of community design that facilitates walking to local destinations).

- Improving pedestrian safety structures, such as traffic lights.

Supporting Discussion

Two published reviews assessed aspects of the built environment and youth activity,[74, 75] although only one[74] focused solely on physical activity in youth and the built environment. One of these was a systematic review of 103 studies that assessed many dimensions of the built environment—both perceived and objective—related to self-reported and objective measures of activity in youth. This review[74] provides the most comprehensive assessment of the built environment and youth activity, and its findings serve as the basis for our conclusions. The other review[75] evaluated interventions or associations with youth activity that included the built environment as one of many possible influences. This review[75] systematically reviewed only prospective studies. Although some intervention studies were included in the reviews, most studies were cross-sectional, as is typical for this emerging field. Traditional research-initiated interventions in the built environment are often extremely difficult to undertake, given time, expense, jurisdiction, and other logistical considerations.

Associations were found between youth activity and traffic-related safety, but not to crime-related safety. However, this may be an artifact of the measures used in studies assessing crime-related safety and youth physical activity, and/or review methodolgy.[74]

These conclusions related to those aspects of the built environment and increased youth activity are largely consistent with findings from literature on youth active transportation and literature on the built environment and the general population.

Camps and Youth Organizations

Communities often offer physical activity opportunities outside of the traditional school setting as part of youth organizations, such as scouting, or places, such as camps. Scouting is defined as activities of various national and international organizations that help youth develop character, citizenship, and individual skills. Camps are defined as places, often in rural areas, used for recreation or instruction and often held during the summer.

Many youth attend camps or scouting activities as part of their participation in community organizations. For example, approximately 5 million youth participate in either the Girls Scouts or Boy Scouts of America.[76, 77] Because of their broad reach, camps and scouting organizations are promising venues by which to improve youth physical activity. Camps and scouting organizations increase youth physical activity through strategies, such as providing opportunities for youth to be active during the camp or scouting experiences, or by creating incentives for physical activity as part of organizational goals or policies. The reviews discussed in this section of the report primarily covered the first strategy.

Supporting Discussion

Three narrative reviews included the summer camp or scouting setting, although no review specifically focused on interventions to increase physical activity in either of these settings.[42, 50, 57] Two of the reviews[42, 50] comprehensively evaluated summer camp or scouting interventions and included a section on physical activity in their conclusions. The third review[57] did not provide summary information about physical activity interventions in the summer camp or scouting setting.

Taken together, the reviews concluded that using summer camp or scouting strategies to increase youth physical activity may be a promising intervention strategy, although its effectiveness has not yet been shown.

In the summer camp setting, physical activity has been promoted along with other strategies, such as Internet-based education.[78] Interventions in Girl

Scouts have successfully used troop leaders to deliver an educational curriculum along with modifications to troop meeting policies and badge assignments to increase physical activity.[79] Interventions conducted as part of scouting or summer camps also have used accelerometry and self-report methods to measure physical activity. These few studies had mixed results, but suggest that this setting may provide promising opportunities for youth to increase physical activity.

Other Community-based Programs

The Guide to Community Preventive Services[67] defines community-based interventions as those "conducted within and by members of a particular community (e.g., grassroots efforts, efforts by a local civic group)." Community-based programs in youth are carried out in diverse settings, including community centers and recreation facilities, churches, housing projects, and school facilities. They are conducted outside of school day hours or on weekends.

Conclusion

Evidence is insufficient that intervention strategies set in the community increase physical activity among youth.

Supporting Discussion

Two systematic reviews,[51, 54] three narrative reviews,[26, 27, 42] and one recent review-of-reviews with an additional literature update[80] included interventions set in the community or in community centers. Two of the narrative reviews[26, 27] also were included in the review-of-reviews. One review focused on studies encompassing a broad definition of community; the remaining five reviews included a small number of studies of broadly defined community interventions as well as school plus community interventions as part of a multi-setting review. No review focused specifically on interventions within community centers.

Few studies included in the six reviews formally examined the association between community-based interventions and youth physical activity. Among those that did, interventions were conducted outside of the school day and in a variety of settings. A mix of intervention strategies were used, including informational sessions, joint-use programs, and after-school activities. The effectiveness of specific intervention strategies was difficult to ascertain because of the diverse array of intervention strategies. Physical activity was assessed using a variety of methods, including direct observation, self-report, pedometers, and accelerometers.

For the most part, the reviews did not provide convincing evidence of a positive effect of community strategies on physical activity in youth. Some evidence suggests that interventions developed in the school setting that include community linkages as part of a comprehensive socio-ecologic approach can increase youth physical activity. However, the findings are limited for adolescents and even more scarce for children. Providing supervised access to school playgrounds during non-school hours also shows promise, as this type of intervention was found to be associated with increased levels of physical activity in a pilot study of inner city elementary school-aged children.

Next Steps for Research in the Community Setting

- Conduct studies with longer intervention periods and long-term follow up.

- Conduct quasi-experimental evaluation research on the built environment and youth physical activity, taking advantage of "natural experiments" (i.e., environmental changes implemented by policymakers and/or others).

- Evaluate effects of built environment changes on adolescent physical activity.

- Assess the effect of neighborhood crime-related safety on youth physical activity.

- Develop methods to improve attendance in the programs and interventions under study.

- Examine ways to convert summer camp activity into habitual activity.

- Examine the role of "location in the community," particularly distance from school or home, on participation and adherence.

- Compare intervention effects across race, ethnicity, and socioeconomic groups.

Family and Home Setting

Physical activity interventions focused on the family and home are designed to improve health-related behaviors and prevent obesity. This setting is logical, given that children develop physical activity behaviors, attitudes, and values in the home.[81] Parents structure much of their children's time during early childhood through adolescence, thus enabling or constraining exposure to physical activities. Parents and other caregivers also influence physical activity behaviors through their control of resources, such as through buying sporting equipment or transporting a child to lessons and sporting activities.

Research addressing physical activity correlates and determinants indicate that parents and other family members are important in explaining differences in physical activity levels among youth.[82] Of critical significance is evidence that physical activity behaviors tend to aggregate within a family. That is, active parents tend to have active children. For example, using objective measures of physical activity, the Framingham Heart Study reported that young children with two active parents were 5.8 times more likely to be active than children with two inactive parents.[83]

Family and home-based interventions can include one or more approaches to support behavioral change, including informational and educational (for parents and children), behavioral and social (exercise or fitness programs), and policy and environmental (family policies for outdoor time, access to equipment). In addition, parents and other family members play important support roles for interventions that primarily take place in settings other than the home, such as schools. Interventions that target the home should reflect the reality that families are complex, dynamic, and encompass a variety of structures and cultures.

Conclusion

Evidence is insufficient that interventions strategies in the family and home increase physical activity among youth.

Supporting Discussion

Few studies have specifically examined the effectiveness of interventions in the family and home setting. Of these few, methodological problems, including the lack of long-term follow-up, poor validity of selected physical activity measures, small study samples, and limited information on intervention fidelity and implementation, hamper clear conclusions.

Three reviews were identified that specifically focused on family and home-based interventions.[80, 84, 85] Sending materials home through newsletters or homework, or by physical activity programs in which parents and children participate together appeared to have no effect. Earlier reviews, which indicated positive effects for increasing physical activity if the interventions were located in the home and included self-monitoring, goal setting, and in-home activities, were not successfully replicated in later research. Although inconclusive, there is some evidence that direct contact with parents may be effective. For example, interventions in which parents are responsible for their children's participation and those in which families are engaged in the intervention through organizations in which they already are involved may be effective.

Next Steps for Research in the Family and Home Setting

- Conduct observational studies to examine the relevance of family and home-based strategies throughout childhood and adolescence.

- Conduct longitudinal, observational studies to delineate which components of family life influence children's physical activity behavior.

- Test specific strategies that engage parents and other family members in promoting physical activity in the home setting.

- Test specific strategies that enrich the home environment to favor activity over sedentary pursuits.

- Compare intervention effects across race, ethnicity, and socioeconomic groups.

Primary Health Care Setting

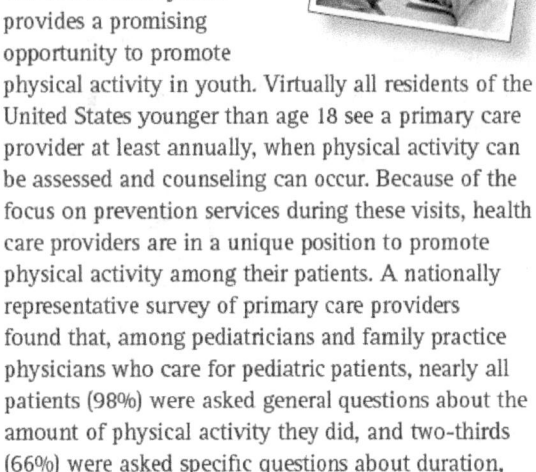

The health care system provides a promising opportunity to promote physical activity in youth. Virtually all residents of the United States younger than age 18 see a primary care provider at least annually, when physical activity can be assessed and counseling can occur. Because of the focus on prevention services during these visits, health care providers are in a unique position to promote physical activity among their patients. A nationally representative survey of primary care providers found that, among pediatricians and family practice physicians who care for pediatric patients, nearly all patients (98%) were asked general questions about the amount of physical activity they did, and two-thirds (66%) were asked specific questions about duration, intensity, and type of physical activity.[86] This suggests that clinicians providing care to pediatric patients may be open to effective counseling interventions. Because of the large number of youth who can be reached, primary care setting interventions could be an efficient mechanism.

Federal and organizational initiatives and recommendations advocate primary care as an appropriate setting for interventions. For example, the Healthy People 2020 objective PA-11.2 is to increase the proportion of physician visits made by all child and adult patients that include counseling about exercise.[45] Starting in 2009, youth physical activity assessment and counseling are measured as part of determining the quality of preventive health care of children and adolescents through the Healthcare Effectiveness Data and Information Set (HEDIS), a tool used by more than 90 percent of America's health systems to measure their quality performance.[87] These policy strategies, along with required measurement indices, indicate a supportive environment for physical activity counseling interventions for youth in the primary care setting. This appeal undoubtedly comes from counseling successes with other health behaviors. For example, the United States Preventive Services Task Force recommends counseling to prevent sexually transmitted infections in "at risk" adolescent populations.[88] Effective strategies in this context were of moderate to high intensity and included individual and group counseling.

Conclusion

Evidence is insufficient that strategies implemented in primary health care settings increase physical activity among youth.

Supporting Discussion

No reviews specifically focusing on the primary care setting were identified, although three included this setting as part of their multi-setting examination of the data.[27, 51, 89] In these reviews, six intervention studies were identified; only one included a control group. Three studies were conducted in Europe and three in the United States. Two studies found no difference in physical activity after a primary care intervention, and four found some increase from baseline, although most measures of physical activity were self-reported and the studies did not report validity and reliability of the physical activity measure. The controlled study did not observe a difference between the intervention and control groups when physical activity was assessed with accelerometers. The studies varied in their approaches so any effective intervention components could not be determined.

The reviews identified a variety of intervention strategies, including brief, extended, or tailored counseling; parental involvement; telephone follow-up; materials sent home; and websites. These components may have been conducted in combination, but little information is available to identify which may be more successful than others. Because of the insufficient information on the validity and reliability of the physical activity assessment methods and the pre-post- study design for most studies, the positive results found in some studies need verification from studies using high-quality study designs. Finally, half of the studies were conducted outside of the United States in countries with different health care systems, which calls into question how replicable potentially effective strategies may be.

Next Steps for Research in the Primary Health Care Setting

- Conduct randomized, controlled studies of the effectiveness of primary care counseling on physical activity behavior.

- Identify the optimal intensity and delivery mode of primary care physical activity interventions.

- Consider the utility of interventions that combine primary care counseling with referral and integration into community youth-focused programs.

- Identify the optimal age range for effective interventions in primary care settings, as well as intervention effects in normal weight as well as overweight or obese youth.

- Examine strategies to promote physical activity in different primary care settings, including integrated health care, fee-for-service, and community clinics.

- Conduct cost-effectiveness research after effective interventions have been identified.

- Compare intervention effects across race, ethnicity, and socioeconomic groups.

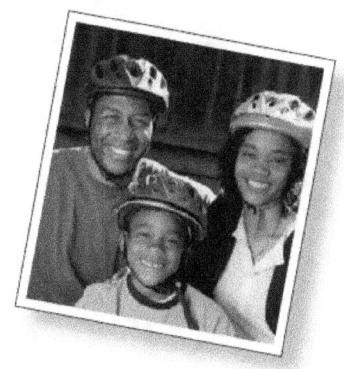

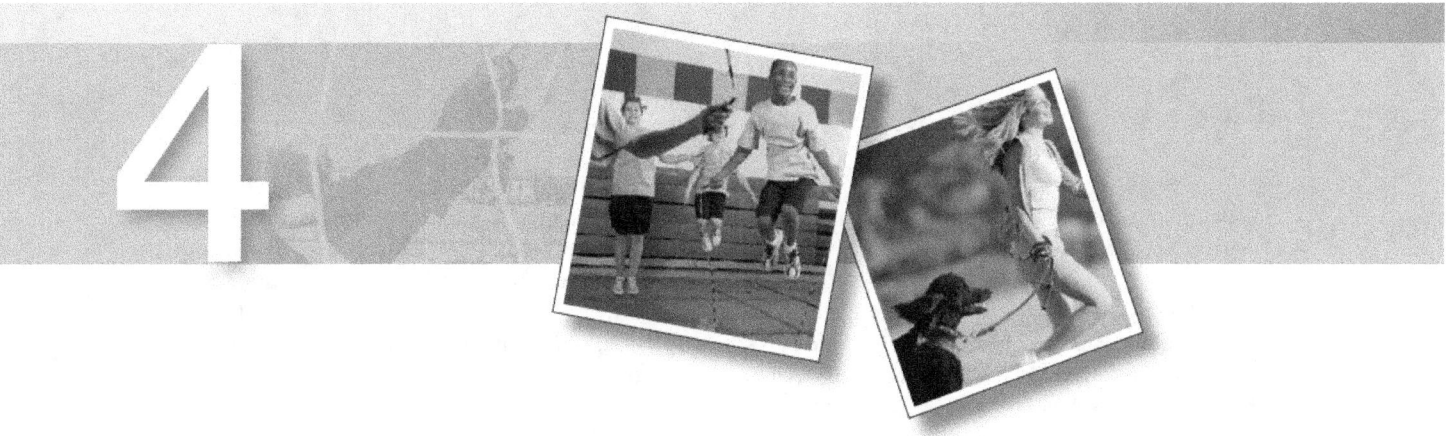

4

Additional Approaches to Consider

The evidence weighed in this *Midcourse Report* includes information from published review articles. As such, some approaches could not be addressed in this review-of-reviews because no reviews have directly addressed the issue or because the approaches are too new to have been attempted very often, too new to have generated a review paper, or underused for other reasons. However, these approaches may be promising for increasing physical activity, and the subcommittee felt it was necessary to identify them as areas for future investigation. These approaches include policy, social marketing, social media and Internet-based approaches, active video games, mobile phones, and outdoor activities.

Policy

Policies and programs can shape environments to promote (or impede) physical activity. They have broad reach across the population and are therefore potentially powerful tools to increase physical activity and fitness. With increased attention on the current and future health of America's youth and efforts like the First Lady Michelle Obama's *Let's Move!* initiative, policy solutions have been recommended.[90-93] Policymakers' interest in youth physical activity has increased, with improved physical activity levels seen as a goal in itself, as well as a component of comprehensive efforts to address rates of childhood obesity.

Policy involvement in youth activity has ample precedent. Two examples stand out in particular:

- PE has been an institution in American schools since the late 19th century, and currently most states mandate PE for students in elementary (84% of states), middle (80%), and high schools (86%). Although the quality and quantity of PE actually provided to U.S. students typically falls below recommended standards, the high prevalence of state-mandated PE constitutes a longstanding, widespread and important policy that directly supports the provision of physical activity to students.[94]

- In 1972, Congress passed and President Nixon signed Title IX of the Education Amendments of 1972. Title IX banned exclusion from educational programs and activities on the basis of gender. Over the following four decades, this legislation has transformed sport participation opportunities for girls and women in American high schools, colleges, and universities. According to the National Federation of State High School Associations, girls' participation in high school sports programs increased from less than 300,000 in 1971–1972 to more than 3.2 million in 2011–2012.[95] Title IX, a policy aimed primarily at addressing gender inequity, has clearly expanded physical activity opportunities tremendously for millions of adolescent girls.

Although individual articles have assessed the implementation and/or content of policies related to youth activity[96-98] as well as associations between different policies with youth activity,[99-101] no extant reviews have directly examined policy and youth physical activity. Nevertheless, it is important to note that policymakers have authority over several of the settings identified in this report as potentially important avenues for increasing youth physical activity, and for which research reviews indicate beneficial effects:

- Schools can influence activity in youth through PE, recess, other activity breaks, active transportation to school, and enhancements to the school environment. Promoting physical activity in schools has traditionally been part of the U.S. education system, and research indicates its beneficial effects on both health and education. A growing body of research addressing the association between physical activity and academic achievement indicates that school-based physical activity can improve grades, standardized test scores, cognitive skills, concentration, and attention. (See the School section of this report for more details, p. 9.)

  Other school-related policies also may increase youth physical activity. Joint- and shared-use agreements—policies that allow youth and other community members to use school physical activity facilities outside school hours[102]—may increase community access to and used of recreation facilities, potentially increasing physical activity levels. In addition, school siting may influence physical activity in youth; research suggests that distance to school is inversely associated with biking or walking to school.[103-105]

- Preschool and Childcare settings appear to be an important venue in which activity levels of young children may be affected. These effects occur through providing portable play equipment on playgrounds and other play spaces, providing staff

with training in delivery of structured physical activity sessions for children and increasing the time allocated for such sessions, integrating physically active teaching and learning activities into pre-academic instructional routines, and increasing time that children spend outside. Policies promoting structured physical activity in childcare should consider the need for teacher training, as research suggests that teachers' knowledge about physical activity, motor development, and their ability to support children's learning and development is important. Physical activity can and should be integrated into the daily routines and existing curricula of preschools, and should not be seen as something that competes with other educational goals. (See the Preschool and Childcare Centers section of this report for more details, p. 15.)

- Aspects of the built environment appear to influence youth activity, specifically those under the jurisdictions of urban planning, transportation, and parks and recreation. Examples include: modifications that encourage active transportation, walking and biking, pedestrian safety, reduced traffic speed and volume, reduced incivilities and disorders (such as litter and vacant lots), and access to, density of, and proximity to places for youth to be active, such as parks and recreation centers. (See the Community section of this report for more details, p. 16.) It is worth noting that policies encouraging increased active transportation among youth—namely, walking or biking to school or other destinations—may have the triple benefit of improving children's cardiometabolic health as well as improving air quality and environmental sustainability.

- Social marketing is another method available to policymakers for increasing physical activity in youth, and research suggests that targeted media campaigns have improved other youth health behaviors, such as smoking.[106, 107] Although results of mass media campaigns to increase physical activity have been mixed,[108] a notable success is the VERB™ campaign, discussed in greater detail on p. 25.

All levels of government are able to play a role in shaping evidence-informed policies and programs to increase youth activity. At the local level, municipal and county governments are responsible for managing the built environment directly, and local school districts influence activity-related policies within their jurisdictions, such as PE requirements. At the state and national level, policymakers can exert substantial influence through legislation, appropriations, and other incentives related to urban planning, transportation, parks and recreation, education, and childcare. Examples include a recent policy change in Massachusetts for minimum activity requirements in childcare, and the national Safe Routes to School program from the U.S. Department of Transportation.[109] It is especially important to engage partners from a variety of sectors in health-related policymaking in the quest to increase physical activity in youth.[110]

VERB™

When planning for strategies to increase physical activity in U.S youth, much can be learned from successes of the past. The VERB campaign is one recent example of a population-based approach that increased physical activity among U.S. youth. The 2001–2006 VERB campaign was a national, multicultural, social marketing campaign coordinated by CDC. Funded at $339 million over 5 years, the mission of VERB was to increase and maintain physical activity among U.S. youth ages 9 to 13 ("tweens"). This age group was selected because of the precipitous decrease in physical activity that occurs during adolescence. Campaign planners made significant efforts to involve tweens themselves and, in fact, the name of the campaign— VERB—and its tagline—It's what you do!™—were chosen because they were the most popular options among participating tweens.

VERB used a social marketing approach in a campaign to deliver a positive and educational message about physical activity through media messages delivered by television, radio, and newspaper advertising; school and community promotions; the Internet; and national and local partnerships. Messages were tailored to reach a general audience of tweens and their parents, as well as specific racial and ethnic groups.[111] To extend its reach, the campaign also engaged other adults with

influence in the life of tweens, such as teachers, youth leaders, PE and health professionals, pediatricians, health care providers, and coaches.

VERB had many successes, demonstrating that a concentrated marketing campaign, with substantial funding and a multi-sector approach, can positively affect physical activity levels in youth. At the end of the first year, nearly three-quarters of tweens surveyed were aware of the campaign, and those who were aware were more likely to report participating in physical activity during their free time than were those who were unaware of the campaign.[111] After 2 years, the program showed a dose-response effect, namely that greater reported frequency of exposure to VERB messages was associated with more reported activity in tweens.[112] Awareness of the VERB campaign remained high over time—three-quarters of tweens were aware of the campaign toward the end of the funding period in 2006, and again, tweens exposed to the campaign were more likely to report being physically active than were those who were unaware of the campaign. Finally, evidence suggests that exposure to VERB during the tween years had carry-over value into adolescence (youth ages 13 to 17). Tweens experiencing greater exposure to VERB reported higher benefits of physical activity and greater amounts of free-time physical activity in later years.[113]

Today's tweens are different from those who originally contributed to the development and successes of VERB. For one thing, in the 10 years since VERB began, the way tweens receive and share information has changed dramatically. A national effort replicating the successful strategies used in the VERB campaign must address today's youth. In order to capitalize on the prior success of VERB, any future physical activity efforts must incorporate technology, social media, and the Internet to an even greater degree than did VERB.

Technology-based Approaches

Social media and Internet-based approaches involve the use of Facebook, Twitter, other similar social media avenues, and websites. The Internet is a major force in societal development that will continue to shape people's lives during the next 10 to 15 years at the global level.[15] Data from the 2010 U.S. Census indicate that 76 percent of U.S. residents ages 3 and older live in a household with Internet access, and 65 percent of residents ages 3 and older access the Internet at home.[114] The Pew Internet Survey reported that 95 percent of youth ages 12 to 17 are Internet users and 80 percent use social media sites.[115] Almost all U.S. children and adolescents can be reached through social media and Internet-based programming. Clearly, children and adolescents are interested in these types of activities, and researchers should continue to explore their potential uses in interventions to increase physical activity.

Children and adolescents are increasingly exposed to new technology that they have embraced. Technology applied to increasing physical activity is a developing strategy with wide open possibilities. For example, active video games ("exergames") and mobile phone technologies have exponentially increased. A 2008 Pew Report noted that 97 percent of youth ages 12 to 17 play video games, with 50 percent reporting they played the previous day.[115] Approximately 86 percent play on some type of console.[115] In a recent review of active video game interventions in children and adults, evidence was not sufficient to suggest that playing active video games increases physical activity. However, technology in this area is rapidly changing, rendering some of the possible reasons for uncertain effects obsolete.[116] For example, platform changes introduced by the video game industry now force players to actually move during games instead of simulating movement with a game controller while sitting.

Mobile phones are another social media and Internet device whose use has skyrocketed in recent years. A July 2011 Pew Internet Survey noted that 77 percent of youth ages 12 to 17 had a mobile phone, and the number of smartphones used in this population is on the increase.[115] Apps are now available that track physical activity. For example, the inclusion of Global Positioning Systems (GPS) and accelerometer technology in mobile phones allows programs to estimate the number of miles walked per day. Children and adolescents are drawn to these types of tools and may increase physical activity just to be able to use the tools for fun.

Playing Outdoors

In addition to these new technologies, some tried-and-true methods have great merit and should continue to be emphasized in future interventions. It may seem intuitive and therefore seldom designated as a specific strategy, but simply getting children and adolescents to spend time outdoors is a simple and low-cost approach for increasing physical activity because almost all outside child and adolescent-appropriate activities encourage some level of physical activity. Several studies have shown, across a wide range of age groups, that spending time outside is associated with increased levels of moderate-to-vigorous intensity physical activity.[117-122] Additionally, studies have shown that dog ownership is related to physical activity among adolescents,[123] suggesting that taking the dog for walks may increase physical activity. In contrast to technology-based activities, which primarily take place indoors, encouraging children to spend time outdoors may provide extra benefit because being physically active outside creates positive feelings about exercise.[124] In addition, some activities that are most easily accommodated in outdoor settings, such as jumping rope, playing hop-scotch, and doing hip hop dance moves, have specific and substantial health benefits, including developing strong bones.[125]

In summary, policy approaches, social marketing, social media and Internet-based approaches, active video games, mobile phones, and outdoor activities all have promise for increasing physical activity in youth, despite the current lack of evidence for employing them. Other strategies not mentioned in this document, such as focusing on social aspects of physical activity, may hold promise as well. The subcommittee recommends creative thinking as we move into the future. It also is important to remember lessons learned, in particular the one from VERB indicating that we should include youth—the primary audience we wish to reach—in designing and implementing physical activity interventions, in order to increase the likelihood of success.

References

1. Synder TD, Dillow SA. Digest of education statistics 2010. Washington, DC: National Center for Education Statistics, Institute of Education Sciences, US Department of Education; 2011.

2. Federal Interagency Forum on Child and Family Statistics. America's children in brief: key national indicators of well-being, 2006. Washington, DC: US Government Printing Office; 2006.

3. Handy SL, Boarnet MG, Ewing R, et al. How the built environment affects physical activity: views from urban planning. Am J Prev Med. 2002; 23(2 Suppl):64-73.

4. Physical Activity Guidelines Advisory Committee. Physical Activity Guidelines Advisory Committee report, 2008. Washington, DC: US Department of Health and Human Services; 2008.

5. May AL, Kuklina EV, Yoon PW. Prevalence of cardiovascular disease risk factors among US adolescents, 1999-2008. Pediatrics. 2012;129(6): 1035-41.

6. Centers for Disease Control and Prevention. The association between school based physical activity, including physical education, and academic performance. Atlanta, GA: US Department of Health and Human Services; July 2010.

7. Centers for Disease Control and Prevention. Youth risk behavior surveillance–United States, 2011. MMWR 2012;61(No. SS-04):1-162.

8. Troiano RP, Berrigan D, Dodd KW, et al. Physical activity in the United States measured by accelerometer. Med Sci Sports Exerc. 2008;40(1): 181-8.

9. US Department of Health and Human Services. 2008 Physical activity guidelines for Americans. Washington, DC: US Department of Health and Human Services; 2008.

10. Institute of Medicine. Committee on Obesity Prevention Policies for Young Children. Early childhood obesity prevention policies. Washington, DC: The National Academies Press; 2011.

11. Pate RR, O'Neill JR. Physical activity guidelines for young children: an emerging consensus. Arch Pediatr Adolesc Med. 2012:1-2.

12. Australian Government, Department of Health and Ageing. National physical activity recommendations for children 0-5 years old. 2010.

13. United Kingdom Department of Health. New physical activity guidelines 2011. Available from: http://www.dh.gov.uk/health/2011/07/ physical-activity-guidelines/.

14. Heath GW, Parra DC, Sarmiento OL, et al. Evidence-based intervention in physical activity: lessons from around the world. Lancet. 2012;380(9838):272-81.

15. Pratt M, Sarmiento OL, Montes F, et al. The implications of megatrends in information and communication technology and transportation for changes in global physical activity. Lancet. 2012;380(9838):282-93.

16. Snyder TD, Dillow SA. Digest of Education Statistics 2011. Washington, DC: National Center for Education Statistics, Institute of Education Sciences, US Department of Education; 2012.

17. Kahn EB, Ramsey LT, Brownson RC, et al. The effectiveness of interventions to increase physical activity. A systematic review. Am J Prev Med. 2002;22(4 Suppl):73-107.

18. Trudeau F, Shephard RJ. Contribution of school programmes to physical activity levels and attitudes in children and adults. Sports Med. 2005;35(2): 89-105.

19. Dale D, Corbin CB. Physical activity participation of high school graduates following exposure to conceptual or traditional physical education. Res Q Exerc Sport. 2000;71(1):61-8.

20. Xiang P, McBride R, Guan J. Children's motivation in elementary physical education: a longitudinal study. Res Q Exerc Sport. 2004;75(1):71-80.

21. Pelligrini AD, Kato K, Blatchford P, Baines E. A short-term longitudinal study of children's playground games across the first year of school: implications for social competence and adjustment to school. Am Educ Res J. 2002;39:991-1015.

22. Hellison D. Physical activity programs for underserved youth. J Sci Med Sport. 2000;3(3): 238-42.

23. Dishman RK, Motl RW, Sallis JF, et al. Self-management strategies mediate self-efficacy and physical activity. Am J Prev Med. 2005;29(1):10-8.

24. Dishman RK, Motl RW, Saunders R, et al. Enjoyment mediates effects of a school-based physical-activity intervention. Med Sci Sports Exerc. 2005;37(3): 478-87.

25. Kriemler S, Meyer U, Martin E, et al. Effect of school-based interventions on physical activity and fitness in children and adolescents: a review of reviews and systematic update. Br J Sports Med. 2011;45(11): 923-30.

26. van Sluijs EM, McMinn AM, Griffin SJ. Effectiveness of interventions to promote physical activity in children and adolescents: systematic review of controlled trials. BMJ. 2007;335(7622):703.

27. Salmon J, Booth ML, Phongsavan P, et al. Promoting physical activity participation among children and adolescents. Epidemiol Rev. 2007;29:144-59.

28. Demetriou Y, Honer O. Physical activity interventions in the school setting a systematic review. Psychol Sport Exerc. 2012;13(2):186-96.

29. Sharma M. Physical activity interventions in Hispanic American girls and women. Obes Rev. 2008;9(6): 560-71.

30. Dobbins M, De Corby K, Robeson P, et al. School-based physical activity programs for promoting physical activity and fitness in children and adolescents aged 6-18. Cochrane Database Syst Rev. 2009(1):CD007651.

31. De Bourdeaudhuij I, Van Cauwenberghe E, Spittaels H, et al. School-based interventions promoting both physical activity and healthy eating in Europe: a systematic review within the HOPE project. Obes Rev. 2011;12(3):205-16.

32. National Association for Sport and Physical Education. Moving into the future: national standards for physical education, 2nd ed. Reston, VA: National Association for Sport and Physical Education; 2004.

33. Sallis JF, McKenzie TL, Alcaraz JE, et al. The effects of a 2-year physical education program (SPARK) on physical activity and fitness in elementary school students. Sports, Play and Active Recreation for Kids. Am J Public Health. 1997;87(8):1328-34.

34. Luepker RV, Perry CL, McKinlay SM, et al. Outcomes of a field trial to improve children's dietary patterns and physical activity. The Child and Adolescent Trial for Cardiovascular Health. CATCH collaborative group. JAMA. 1996;275(10):768-76.

35. Donnelly JE, Jacobsen DJ, Whatley JE, et al. Nutrition and physical activity program to attenuate obesity and promote physical and metabolic fitness in elementary school children. Obes Res. 1996;4(3): 229-43.

36. McKenzie TL, Marshall SJ, Sallis JF, et al. Student activity levels, lesson context, and teacher behavior during middle school physical education. Res Q Exerc Sport. 2000;71(3):249-59.

37. McKenzie TL, Nader PR, Strikmiller PK, et al. School physical education: effect of the Child and Adolescent Trial for Cardiovascular Health. Prev Med. 1996;25(4):423-31.

38. Pate RR, Ward DS, Saunders RP, et al. Promotion of physical activity among high-school girls: a randomized controlled trial. Am J Public Health. 2005;95(9):1582-7.

39. Slingerland M, Borghouts L. Direct and indirect influence of physical education-based interventions on physical activity: a review. J Phys Act Health. 2011;8(6):866-78.

40. Khan LK, Sobush K, Keener D, et al. Recommended community strategies and measurements to prevent obesity in the United States. MMWR Recomm Rep. 2009 Jul 24;58(RR-7):1-26.

41. Hoehner CM, Soares J, Parra Perez D, et al. Physical activity interventions in Latin America: a systematic review. Am J Prev Med. 2008;34(3):224-33.

42. Camacho-Minano MJ, LaVoi NM, Barr-Anderson DJ. Interventions to promote physical activity amoung young and adolescent girls: a systematic review. Health Educ Res. 2011;26(6):1025-49.

43. Chillon P, Evenson KR, Vaughn A, et al. A systematic review of interventions for promoting active transportation to school. Int J Behav Nutr Phys Act. 2011;8:10.

44. McDonald NC. Active transportation to school: trends among U.S. schoolchildren, 1969-2001. Am J Prev Med. 2007;32(6):509-16.

45. US Department of Health and Human Services. Healthy People 2020. Physical activity objectives. Washington, DC; 2012 [cited 2012 September 17]. Available from: http://www.healthypeople.gov/2020/topicsobjectives2020/objectiveslist.aspx?topicId=33.

46. Lee MC, Orenstein MR, Richardson MJ. Systematic review of active commuting to school and childrens physical activity and weight. J PhysAct Health. 2008;5(6):930-49.

47. Faulkner GE, Buliung RN, Flora PK, et al. Active school transport, physical activity levels and body weight of children and youth: a systematic review. Prev Med. 2009;48(1):3-8.

48. Pucher J, Dill J, Handy S. Infrastructure, programs, and policies to increase bicycling: an international review. Prev Med. 2010;50 Suppl 1:S106-25.

49. Ogilvie D, Foster CE, Rothnie H, et al. Interventions to promote walking: systematic review. BMJ. 2007;334(7605):1204.

50. Jago R, Baranowski T. Non-curricular approaches for increasing physical activity in youth: a review. Prev Med. 2004;39(1):157-63.

51. De Meester F, van Lenthe FJ, Spittaels H, et al. Interventions for promoting physical activity among European teenagers: a systematic review. Int J Behav Nutr Phys Act. 2009;6:82.

52. van Stralen MM, Yildirim M, te Velde SJ, et al. What works in school-based energy balance behaviour interventions and what does not? A systematic review of mediating mechanisms. Int J Obes. 2011;35(10):1251-65.

53. Harrison F, Jones AP. A framework for understanding school based physical environmental influences on childhood obesity. Health Place. 2012;18(3):639-48.

54. Atkin AJ, Gorely T, Biddle SJ, et al. Interventions to promote physical activity in young people conducted in the hours immediately after school: a systematic review. Int J Behav Med. 2011;18(3):176-87.

55. Pate RR, O'Neill JR. After-school interventions to increase physical activity among youth. Br J Sports Med. 2009;43(1):14-8.

56. Beets MW, Beighle A, Erwin HE, et al. After-school program impact on physical activity and fitness: a meta-analysis. Am J Prev Med. 2009;36(6):527-37.

57. Timperio A, Salmon J, Ball K. Evidence-based strategies to promote physical activity among children, adolescents and young adults: review and update. J Sci Med Sport. 2004;7(1 Suppl):20-9.

58. Dowda M, Pate RR, Trost SG, et al. Influences of preschool policies and practices on children's physical activity. J Community Health. 2004;29(3):183-96.

59. Bower JK, Hales DP, Tate DF, et al. The childcare environment and children's physical activity. Am J Prev Med. 2008;34(1):23-9.

60. Dowda M, Brown WH, McIver KL, et al. Policies and characteristics of the preschool environment and physical activity of young children. Pediatrics. 2009;123(2):e261-6.

61. Boldemann C, Blennow M, Dal H, et al. Impact of preschool environment upon children's physical activity and sun exposure. Prev Med. 2006;42(4):301-8.

62. Brown WH, Pfeiffer KA, McIver KL, et al. Social and environmental factors associated with preschoolers' nonsedentary physical activity. Child Dev. 2009;80(1):45-58.

63. Cardon G, Van Cauwenberghe E, Labarque V, et al. The contribution of preschool playground factors in explaining children's physical activity during recess. Int J Behav Nutr Phys Act. 2008;5:11.

64. Kreichauf S, Wildgruber A, Krombholz H, et al. Critical narrative review to identify educational strategies promoting physical activity in preschool. Obes Rev. 2012;13 Suppl 1:96-105.

65. Nixon CA, Moore HJ, Douthwaite W, et al. Identifying effective behavioural models and behaviour change strategies underpinning preschool- and school-based obesity prevention interventions aimed at 4-6-year-olds: a systematic review. Obes Rev. 2012;13 Suppl 1:106-17.

66. Ward DS, Vaughn A, McWilliams C, et al. Interventions for increasing physical activity at child care. Med Sci Sports Exerc. 2010;42(3):526-34.

67. Guide to Community Preventive Services. Environmental and policy approaches to increase physical activity: community-scale urban design land use policies, 2004 [cited 2012 October 15]. Available from: http://www.thecommunityguide.org/pa/environmental-policy/communitypolicies.html.

68. Davison KK, Werder JL, Lawson CT. Children's active commuting to school: current knowledge and future directions. Prev Chronic Disease. 2008;5(3):A100.

69. Frank L, Kavage S. A national plan for physical activity: the enabling role of the built environment. J Phys Act Health. 2009;6 Suppl 2:S186-95.

70. Heath GW, Brownson RC, Kruger J, et al. The effectiveness of urban design and land use and transport policies and practices to increase physical activity: a systematic review. J Phys Act Health. 2006;3(Suppl 1):S55-76.

71. Mowen AJ, Baker BL. Park, recreation, fitness, and sport sector recommendations for a more physically active America: a white paper for the United States national physical activity plan. J Phys Act Health. 2009;6 Suppl 2:S236-44.

72. Institute of Medicine (IOM). Local government actions to prevent childhood obesity. Washington, DC: The National Academies Press; 2009.

73. de Vet E, de Ridder DT, de Wit JB. Environmental correlates of physical activity and dietary behaviours among young people: a systematic review of reviews. Obes Rev. 2011;12(5):e130-42.

74. Ding D, Sallis JF, Kerr J, et al. Neighborhood environment and physical activity among youth a review. Am J Prev Med. 2011;41(4):442-55.

75. Craggs C, Corder K, van Sluijs EM, et al. Determinants of change in physical activity in children and adolescents: a systematic review. Am J Prev Med. 2011;40(6):645-58.

76. Girl Scouts. About Girl Scouts of the USA [cited 2012 October 23]. Available from: http://www.girlscouts.org/who_we_are/facts/.

77. Boy Scouts of America. Overiview of Boy Scouts of America [cited 2012 October 23]. Available from: http://www.scouting.org/About/FactSheets/OverviewofBSA.aspx.

78. Baranowski T, Baranowski JC, Cullen KW, et al. The Fun, Food, and Fitness Project (FFFP): the Baylor GEMS pilot study. Ethn Dis. 2003;13(1 Suppl 1): S30-9.

79. Rosenkranz RR, Behrens TK, Dzewaltowski DA. A group-randomized controlled trial for health promotion in Girl Scouts: healthier troops in a SNAP (Scouting Nutrition & Activity Program). BMC Public Health. 2010;10:81.

80. van Sluijs EM, Kriemler S, McMinn AM. The effect of community and family interventions on young people's physical activity levels: a review of reviews and updated systematic review. Br J Sports Med. 2011;45(11):914-22.

81. Brustad R. The role of family in promoting physical activity. Pres Counc Phys Fit Sports Res Dig. 2010 Mar;Series 10(3).

82. Hinkley T, Crawford D, Salmon J, et al. Preschool children and physical activity: a review of correlates. Am J Prev Med. 2008;34(5):435-41.

83. Moore LL, Lombardi DA, White MJ, et al. Influence of parents' physical activity levels on activity levels of young children. J Pediatr. 1991;118(2):215-9.

84. Golley RK, Hendrie GA, Slater A, et al. Interventions that involve parents to improve children's weight-related nutrition intake and activity patterns—what nutrition and activity targets and behaviour change techniques are associated with intervention effectiveness? Obes Rev. 2011;12(2):114-30.

85. O'Connor TM, Jago R, Baranowski T. Engaging parents to increase youth physical activity a systematic review. Am J Prev Med. 2009;37(2):141-9.

86. Huang TT, Borowski LA, Liu B, et al. Pediatricians' and family physicians' weight-related care of children in the U.S. Am J Prev Med. 2011;41(1):24-32.

87. National Committee for Quality Assurance. Healthcare Effectiveness Data and Information Set (HEDIS) 2009, Volume 2. Technical Specifications for Health Plans. Appendix 1—HEDIS 2009 Summary Table of Measures, Product Lines and Changes. Available from: http://www.ncqa.org/Portals/0/HEDISQM/HEDIS2009/2009_Measures.pdf

88. Lin JS, Whitlock E, O'Connor E, et al. Behavioral counseling to prevent sexually transmitted infections: a systematic review for the U.S. Preventive Services Task Force. Ann Intern Med. 2008;149(7):497-508, W96-9.

89. Campbell KJ, Hesketh KD. Strategies which aim to positively impact on weight, physical activity, diet and sedentary behaviours in children from zero to five years. A systematic review of the literature. Obes Rev. 2007;8(4):327-38.

90. Institute of Medicine. Accelerating progress in obesity prevention: solving the weight of the nation. Washington, DC: The National Academies Press; 2012.

91. Institute of Medicine and National Research Council. Local government actions to prevent childhood obesity. Washington, DC: The National Academies Press; 2009.

92. Institute of Medicine. Preventing childhood obesity: health in the balance. Washington, DC: The National Academies Press; 2004.

93. Coordinating Committee and Working Groups for the Physical Activity Plan. The U.S. National Physical Activity Plan 2010 [cited December 6, 2012]. Available from: http://www.physicalactivityplan.org/

94. National Association for Sport and Physical Education and American Heart Association. 2012 Shape of the nation report: status of physical education in the USA. Reston, VA: American Alliance for Health, Physical Education, Recreation, and Dance; 2012.

95. National Women's Law Center. The next generation of Title IX: athletics. Washington, DC,: National Women's Law Center; June 2012. Available from: http://www.nwlc.org/sites/default/files/pdfs/nwlcathletics_titleixfactsheet.pdf.

96. Slater SJ, Nicholson L, Chriqui J, et al. The impact of state laws and district policies on physical education and recess practices in a nationally representative sample of US public elementary schools. Arch Pediatr Adolesc Med. 2012;166(4):311-6.

97. Eyler AA, Brownson RC, Aytur SA, et al. Examination of trends and evidence-based elements in state physical education legislation: a content analysis. J Sch Health. 2010;80(7):326-32.

98. Eyler AA, Swaller EM. An analysis of community use policies in Missouri school districts. J Sch Health. 2012;82(4):175-9.

99. Chriqui JF, Taber DR, Slater SJ, et al. The impact of state safe routes to school-related laws on active travel to school policies and practices in U.S. elementary schools. Health Place. 2012;18(1):8-15.

100. Boarnet MG, Anderson CL, Day K, et al. Evaluation of the California Safe Routes to School legislation: urban form changes and children's active transportation to school. Am J Prev Med. 2005; 28(2 Suppl 2):134-40.

101. Sanchez-Vaznaugh EV, Sanchez BN, Rosas LG, et al. Physical education policy compliance and children's physical fitness. Am J Prev Med. 2012;42(5):452-9.

102. Spengler JD, Young SJ, Linton LS. Schools as a community resource for physical activity: legal considerations for decision makers. Am J Health Promot. 2007;21(4s):390-6.

103. US Environmental Protection Agency. School siting guidelines. Washington, DC: US Environmental Protection Agency; 2011.

104. Larsen K, Gilliland J, Hess P, et al. The influence of the physical environment and sociodemographic characteristics on children's mode of travel to and from school. Am J Public Health. 2009;99(3):520-6.

105. American Academy of Pediatrics Committee on Environmental Health. The built environment: designing communities to promote physical activity in children. Pediatrics. 2009;123(6):1591-8.

106. Siegel M, Biener L. The impact of an antismoking media campaign on progression to established smoking: results of a longitudinal youth study. Am J Public Health. 2000;90(3):380-6.

107. Farrelly MC, Davis KC, Haviland ML, et al. Evidence of a dose-response relationship between "truth" antismoking ads and youth smoking prevalence. Am J Public Health. 2005;95(3):425-31.

108. Brown DR, Soares J, Epping JM, et al. Stand-alone mass media campaigns to increase physical activity: a community guide updated review. Am J Prev Med. 2012;43(5):551-61.

109. US Department of Transportation, Federal Highway Adminstration. Safe routes to school. [cited 2012 October 18]. Available from: http://safety.fhwa.dot.gov/saferoutes/.

110. McKinnon RA, Bowles HR, Trowbridge MJ. Engaging physical activity policymakers. J Phys Act Health. 2011;8 Suppl 1:S145-7.

111. Huhman M, Potter LD, Wong FL, et al. Effects of a mass media campaign to increase physical activity among children: year-1 results of the VERB campaign. Pediatrics. 2005;116(2):e277-84.

112. Huhman ME, Potter LD, Duke JC, et al. Evaluation of a national physical activity intervention for children: VERB campaign, 2002-2004. Am J Prev Med. 2007;32(1):38-43.

113. Huhman ME, Potter LD, Nolin MJ, et al. The Influence of the VERB campaign on children's physical activity in 2002 to 2006. Am J Public Health. 2010;100(4):638-45.

114. US Census Bureau. Computer and Internet use in the United States: 2010: Table 1B. Method of accessing Internet at home for households, by selected householder characteristics: 2010 [cited 2012 October 24]. Available from: http://www.census.gov/hhes/computer/publications/2010.html.

115. Pew Internet and American Life Project. Pew Internet survey: teens [updated April 27, 2012; cited 2012 October 25]. Available from: http://pewinternet.org/Commentary/2012/April/Pew-Internet-Teens.aspx.

116. Peng W, Crouse JC, Lin JH. Using active video games for physical activity promotion: a systematic review of the current state of research. Health Educ Behav. 2012.

117. Klesges RC, Eck LH, Hanson CL, et al. Effects of obesity, social interactions, and physical environment on physical activity in preschoolers. Health Psychol. 1990;9(4):435-49.

118. Sallis JF, Nader PR, Broyles SL, et al. Correlates of physical activity at home in Mexican-American and Anglo-American preschool children. Health Psychol. 1993;12(5):390-8.

119. Baranowski T, Thompson WO, DuRant RH, et al. Observations on physical activity in physical locations: age, gender, ethnicity, and month effects. Res Q Exerc Sport. 1993;64(2):127-33.

120. Cleland V, Crawford D, Baur LA, et al. A prospective examination of children's time spent outdoors, objectively measured physical activity and overweight. Int J Obes (Lond). 2008;32(11):1685-93.

121. Raustorp A, Pagels P, Boldemann C, et al. Accelerometer measured level of physical activity indoors and outdoors during preschool time in Sweden and the United States. J Phys Act Health. 2012;9(6):801-8.

122. Conrad A, Seiwert M, Hunken A, et al. The German Environmental Survey for Children (GerES IV): Reference values and distributions for time-location patterns of German children. Int J Hyg Environ Health. 2012.

123. Sirard JR, Patnode CD, Hearst MO, et al. Dog ownership and adolescent physical activity. Am J Prev Med. 2011;40(3):334-7.

124. Focht BC. Brief walks in outdoor and laboratory environments: effects on affective responses, enjoyment, and intentions to walk for exercise. Res Q Exerc Sport. 2009;80(3):611-20.

125. Gunter KB, Almstedt HC, Janz KF. Physical activity in childhood may be the key to optimizing lifespan skeletal health. Exerc Sport Sci Rev. 2012;40(1):13-21.

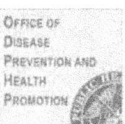
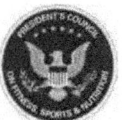

You can find more information about physical activity at:
www.health.gov/paguidelines.

ODPHP Publication No. U0057
December 2012